T0261483

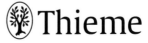

Imaging for Otolaryngologists

Erwin A. Dunnebier, MD, PhD

ENT Surgeon, Otology and Skull Base Surgery
Zaans Medical Center
Zaandam, The Netherlands

In collaboration with:

Erik Beek, MD, PhD
Radiologist
University Medical Center Utrecht
and Wilhelmina Children's Hospital
Utrecht, The Netherlands

Frank Pameijer, MD, PhD
Radiologist
University Medical Center Utrecht
Utrecht, The Netherlands

469 illustrations

Georg Thieme Verlag
Stuttgart · New York

Library of Congress Cataloging-in-Publication Data is available from the publisher.

1st Dutch edition 2007
2nd revised Dutch edition 2007

© Copyright for the Dutch editions remains with the author.

© 2011 Georg Thieme Verlag,
Rüdigerstrasse 14, 70469 Stuttgart, Germany
http://www.thieme.de
Thieme New York, 333 Seventh Avenue,
New York, NY 10001, USA
http://www.thieme.com

Cover design: Thieme Publishing Group
Typesetting by Ziegler & Müller,
Kirchentellinsfurt, Germany
Printed in China by Everbest Printing Ltd

ISBN 978-3-13-146331-9

1 2 3 4 5 6

*To my wife Joyce, and sons Laurens and Florian,
who sacrificed so many moments for the benefit of this book.*

Carpe Momentum

Preface

This book was conceptualized to address the need for a pragmatic and complete overview of radiologic anatomy of the head and neck. Although some aspects of radiologic anatomy are described in extended handbooks of radiology, a step-by-step manual to aid recognition of the normal structures in the entire head and neck region has not been available before.

This book is an illustrated guide to radiologic anatomy of the head and neck as visualized on the most frequently used radiologic modalities, that is, conventional radiography, computed tomography (CT), and magnetic resonance imaging (MRI). Furthermore, radiologic features of the most commonly occurring and characteristic pathologies of the head and neck region are shown, with the aim of aiding recognition earlier in the diagnostic pathway. The differential diagnosis and possible points of interest are also discussed. For MRI, Chapter 1 provides an overview of the interpretation of findings.

For residents, knowledge of normal radiologic anatomy is a first step in recognizing pathology in this field, diagnosing diseases, and planning surgical procedures. For specialists, this book provides an opportunity to update their knowledge and refine their radiologic diagnostic skills in a time of rapidly progressing radiologic techniques.

Most radiologic books are mainly or exclusively written by radiologists. This guide has been designed from the perspective of the field of otorhinolaryngology and will be a vital diagnostic tool in clinical practice. It emphasizes the importance of the relation between clinical features and radiologic findings in the establishment of the correct diagnosis.

Erwin A. Dunnebier

The author welcomes suggestions for improving the content of this book in future editions. If you have any comments, please send an email to dunnebier@zonnet.nl.

Acknowledgements

During my working years at the University Medical Center Utrecht and Wilhelmina Children's Hospital, staff members and residents of the Department of Otorhinolaryngology contributed many of the figures of special cases presented in this book.

Special thanks go to the following:

Erik Beek and Frank Pameijer, radiologists at the University Medical Center Utrecht and Wilhelmina Children's Hospital, The Netherlands. Their contribution in correcting the proofs of the Dutch and English versions symbolizes the symbiotic and complementary relationship between the radiologists and otolaryngologists. Their educational capacities and special interest in otology and the head/neck region highly enriched the interpretation of the figures and the considerations in the differential diagnosis.

Frans Albers, Professor and former Head of the Department of Otolaryngology of the University Medical Center Utrecht, The Netherlands, for his corrections to Chapters 2–5 of the first Dutch edition in his capacity as a neurotologist. Our thanks go to him and his highly motivating skills, which, unfortunately, we miss nowadays.

Gerrit-Jan Hordijk, Professor Emeritus and Head of Department of Otolaryngology of the University Medical Center Utrecht, The Netherlands, for his corrections to Chapters 8 and 9 in his capacity as a head and neck specialist.

Ranny van Weissenbruch, ENT surgeon, specialized in rhinology at the Wilhelmina Hospital Assen, The Netherlands, for his corrections to Chapters 6 and 7 of the English edition.

Furthermore:

Joeri Buwalda, for his corrections to Chapters 6 and 7 of the first Dutch edition.

Anne Schilder, not only for contributing special cases, but also for her motivating personality.

Jos van Overbeek for his active contribution on the subject of radiology of swallowing disorders.

Gérard de Kort, interventional radiologist, for his contribution to this edition.

Contents

General

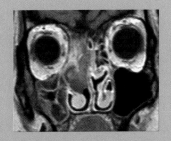

1 Radiographic Imaging Techniques and Interpretation

For the evaluation of sinonasal pathology, conventional radiography (plain films) is still a fast and frequently used tool. However, for more accurate evaluation, computed tomography (CT) and magnetic resonance imaging (MRI) are the modalities of choice. These modalities provide much more information about the localization of pathology, its relation to adjacent structures, and expansive or infiltrative characteristics—factors that play an important role in therapeutic decisions and in planning surgery.

With CT, the bony structures can be well evaluated, especially when evaluating bony outlines. Different settings focusing on bone or soft tissues, as well as the use of contrast agents, can refine the differential diagnosis. Using MRI and its different sequences, characteristics of soft tissues as well as any extension into adjacent structures can be well assessed. The relevant differences between CT and MRI are summarized in **Table 1.1**. For a more extended discussion of the physical characteristics of CT and MRI, as well as their differences, the reader is referred to other manuals listed at the end of this book.

Differentiating Characteristics on CT and MRI

For a detailed evaluation of fine structures on CT, slice thickness and CT settings, as well as the use of intravenous contrast, are important. **Figure 1.1** shows an intraorbitally located subperiosteal abscess resulting from ethmoiditis. The intraorbital abscess may well be missed in the bone setting of **Fig. 1.1a**, since differences between the soft tissues are displayed poorly with contrast, even with the use of intravenous contrast as in this image.

As well as the parameters mentioned for the evaluation of CT, such as slice thickness and use of contrast, tissue differentiation on MRI can be refined by the choice of pulse sequence. In general, interpretation of the most frequently used modality, the turbo spin-echo shown in **Table 1.2**, is of practical value. For a more specific classification and other modalities of MRI, the reader is referred to other manuals or their own department protocol.

Figure 1.2a, b illustrates the complementary tissue differentiation by the two modalities of the same tissue slice in a patient with a T4N0 sinonasal carcinoma.

Table 1.1 Practical differences between CT and MRI

Computed tomography	Magnetic resonance imaging
Utilizes radiation with its inherent danger of oncogenic potency, and potential to damage the eye lens and thyroid gland	Does not require radiation, but there is sometimes a slight local rise of tissue temperature
Fast, widely available	Time-consuming, less widely available
Axial slices, with the possibility of coronal and sagittal reconstructions	Original slices in all directions
Gray values represent the degree of radio-absorption	The degree of resonance is defined by the magnetic strength (Tesla)
The choice of a point of reference defines the setting (bony or soft tissues) and determines the differentiation of tissues	The final image depends on the relaxation times (T1, T2), proton density, flow, and choice of pulses, resulting in more accurate tissue differentiation
Particularly good for the evaluation of bony outlines and structures in relation to air and soft tissues. Differentiation between soft tissues is less accurate	Less suitable for evaluation of bony structures. Accurate evaluation and differentiation of soft tissues as well as their invasive or infiltrative characteristics, also in the area of the skull base
Fewer motion artifacts but strong imaging artifacts related to presence of metals. Metals are not contraindicated	High noise level and patient anxiety in the closed MRI environment may result in artifacts. Magnetic implants might be a contra-indication for MRI due to the danger of dislocation and resulting tissue damage
Risk of allergy to iodinated contrast agents	Allergy to gadolinium is extremely rare

Table 1.2 MRI pulse sequences and tissue differentiation

Tissue	T1-weighted	T2-weighted	T1-weighted gadolinium-enhanced
Water	Hypointense	Strongly hyperintense	Hypointense
Fat	Hyperintense	Hyperintense	Hyperintense
Watery mucus	Hypointense	Hyperintense	Hypointense
Protein-rich mucus	Hyperintense	Hyperintense	Hyperintense
Concentrated mucus	Hypointense	Hypointense	Hypointense
Tumor	Medium (as muscle)	Hyperintense	Hyperintense
Air and bone	No signal	No signal	No signal/hypointense

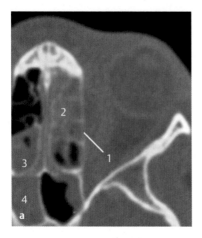

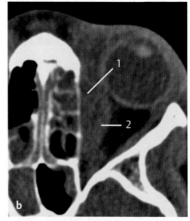

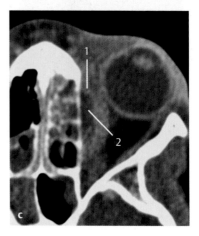

Fig. 1.1 a–c   Axial CT slices of the same level at different settings.

a The bone setting shows an intact lamina papyracea (1) with opacification of the left anterior ethmoid (2), right posterior ethmoid (3), and right sphenoid (4) sinuses.

b Soft-tissue setting without contrast indicates an intraorbital pathology of undetermined nature along the lateral side of the lamina papyracea (1), compressing the medial rectus muscle (2).

c Administration of intravenous contrast shows an abscess with characteristic enhancement of the capsule (1) as well as the abscess contents (2), which are suggestive of fluid.

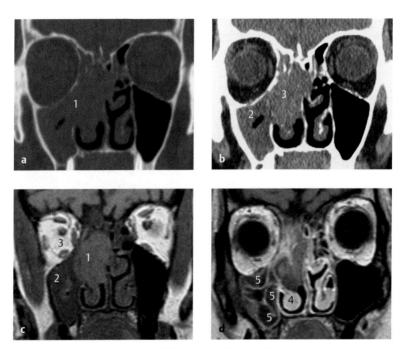

Fig. 1.2 a–e   Differences in tissue differentiation by CT and MRI.

a Coronal CT scan with bone setting shows opacification of the right maxillary sinus and upper part of the intranasal lumen (1). The destruction of the ethmoid cells and medial maxillary wall is well visualized. The lamina papyracea seems intact.

b CT scan with soft-tissue setting shows some differentiation between the contents of the maxillary sinus (2) and the intranasal lumen (3). Intravenous contrast may show a higher degree of differentiation but, in most cases, this is not a regular procedure because of the high cost of contrast agents and possible complications.

c On an unenhanced coronal T1-weighted image, this differentiation is much clearer, with the tumor confined to the intranasal structures and lumen (1). The contents of the maxillary sinus are hypointense (2), and consist of retention cysts or retention of mucus due to obstruction of the maxillary ostium. No invasion of the intraorbital lumen is observed, as demonstrated by an unaffected hyperintense intraorbital fat signal (3).

d The T1-weighted image with gadolinium enhancement shows heterogeneous enhancement of the tumor, with a clear margin to the unaffected inferior turbinate (4). The maxillary content consists of three hypointense (cystic) structures with rim enhancement (5), suggestive of retention cysts.

Fig. 1.2e ▷

Fig. 1.2e

e Axial T2-weighted image at the level of the cranial part of the maxillary sinus. This T2-setting enables differentiation between the tumor, showing medium intensity (1), and the cystic structures, showing a hyper-intense signal (2), confirming the presence of retention cysts with watery content in the maxillary sinus. The air in the left maxillary sinus is visualized as black on all images.

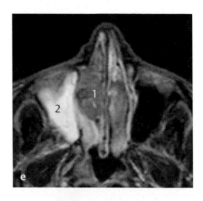

MRI Characteristics of Head and Neck Pathology

Table 1.3 lists the characteristics at presentation of the most frequently observed ENT pathology on different MRI sequences.

Interventional Radiology

Some comments are merited on the growing importance of interventional radiology in the field of otolaryngology. Interventional radiology can be of great help, both in elective procedures and in emergency interventions.

Elective procedures consist mainly of stenting procedures of stenosed or partly occluded vessels in the neck region, as well as embolization of feeding vessels of highly vascularized tumors to reduce intraoperative bleeding. Emergency procedures include treatment of uncontrollable epistaxis or acute embolization of bleeding vessels in the neck, which have been eroded by tumor growth or an abscess. However, not all vessels are easily accessible or can be occluded successfully. Also, complications of the invasive procedure itself, occlusion effects in the devascularized region, or unintended spread of thrombotic occlusive material to other regions of the body have to be taken into account.

Figure 1.3 demonstrates a patient in whom a large laryngeal carcinoma and lymph nodes metastases were removed surgically. Postoperatively, wound healing problems and abscesses probably affected the origin of the external carotid artery, which demonstrates a false aneurysm with extravasation (**Fig. 1.3 a**). Surgical control of the bleeding was difficult to achieve and the interventional radiologist succeeded in occluding the artery (**Fig. 1.3 b**).

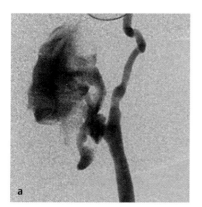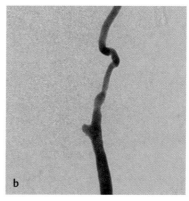

Fig. 1.3 a, b Angiography, anterior views. Control of bleeding after removal of a large laryngeal carcinoma and lymph node metastases. See text for details.

Table 1.3   MRI presentation of common head and neck pathology

Diagnosis (in alphabetical order)	T1-weighted	T2-weighted	T1-weighted, gadolinium-enhanced
Abscess	↓	↑	+ capsule
Adenoid cystic carcinoma	→	→ ↑	+
Aneurysm	Flow voids	Flow voids	+ in case of thrombus
Arachnoidal cyst	↓	↑, isointense to CSF	–
Arteriovenous malformation, dural	Flow voids	Flow voids	+ in case of thrombus or bleeding
Bone marrow	↑	↓	Note: bone is black
Branchial cleft cyst	↓, slightly hyper-intense if infected	↑	Thin wall, thickened wall after infection
Carcinoma, sinonasal	↓ →	→ ↑ hetero-geneous	+ in case of neuronal growth
Cerebral infarction	↓	↑	
Cholesteatoma	↓ →	→ ↑	Sometimes capsule +
Cholesterol granuloma	↑	↑ (capsule ↓)	Sometimes capsule +
Chondrosarcoma	→	↑, voids due to calcifications	+ heterogeneous
Chordoma	↓ → hetero-geneous	↑	+ heterogeneous
Demyelinization	↓ →	↑	+ in case of activity
Dermoid	↑ → ↓	↓ → ↑	–
Effusion, serous stasis	↓	↑	+ in case of granula-tions
Endolymphatic sac tumor	↓ →	→ ↑	+ heterogeneous
Epidermoid cyst	↓ → cholesterol ↑	↑ isointense to CSF	–
Esthesioneuro-blastoma	↓ →	→ ↑ hetero-geneous	+ heterogeneous

Table 1.3 MRI presentation of common head and neck pathology (cont.)

Diagnosis (in alphabetical order)	T1-weighted	T2-weighted	T1-weighted, gadolinium-enhanced
Fibrous dysplasia	↓ → hetero-geneous	↓ → ↑ hetero-geneous	
Glioblastoma	↓ → ↑	↑ heterogeneous	+ edema
Granulations	→	↑	+
Hemangioblastoma	→ sometimes cystic	→ ↑ flow voids	+
Hemangioma	↓ isointense to muscle	↑ heterogeneous	++
Hemangioma, cavernous	↓ not sharply demarcated	↑	+ sometimes thrombosed
Hemangiopericytoma	→	→ (↑)	++
Hematoma • Acute • Subacute • Chronic	 ↓ ↑ ↓ ↑	 ↓ ↓ ↑ 	±/heterogeneous
Hypophysis, adenoma	→ isointense to gray brain	→	+
Juvenile angiofibroma	→	↑ flow voids	++
Labyrinth, hematoma	↑	↑	+
Labyrinthitis	↑	Slightly hyperintense	+
Lipoma	↑ isointense to fat	↓ isointense to fat	–
Lymphadenitis	↓	↑, ↓ in case of abcess	+
Lymphangioma, hygroma colli	↓ ↑	↑ ↑, septal structures ↓	+ multilobular, cystic
Lymphoma, cerebral	Isointense to gray brain	Isointense to gray brain	+ variable
Meningioma	→	→ (↑)	++
Meningitis	↓ →	→ ↑	+ + often also subarachnoidal

Continued on next page

Table 1.3   MRI presentation of common head and neck pathology (cont.)

Diagnosis (in alphabetical order)	T1-weighted	T2-weighted	T1-weighted, gadolinium-enhanced
Metastasis	↓ →	→ ↑	+
Mucocele	↓ watery content or concentrated ↑ proteinaceous	↓ concentrated ↑ watery content or proteinaceous	+ capsule, proteinaceous contents
Orbit, abcess	↓	↑ voids	+ capsule
Orbit, cellulitis	↓	↑	+
Osteomyelitis	↓	↑	+ heterogeneous
Paraganglioma	↓ → isointense to gray brain	→ heterogeneous, flow voids	++
Parotid, Warthin tumor	↓	↑	+ noncystic parts
Parotitis, chronic	↓	↑	+ chronic, ++ acute
Petrositis	↓ →	↑	+ heterogeneous
Pleomorphic adenoma	↓ (↑ hematoma)	↑ (↓ capsule)	+ moderate
Polyposis	↓	↑ ↑	
Retention cyst	↓	↑ ↑	
Rhabdomyosarcoma	↓	↑	+ variable
Sarcoidosis	↓ →	→ ↑	+ nodular and meningeal
Schwannoma	↓ →	→ ↑	++
Sialadenosis	↓ fibrosis ↑ fat	↓ fibrosis ↑ fat	
Sinusitis	↓ (↑ protein)	↑ (↓ protein)	
Sinusitis, fungal	↓	↓	Voids in case of concrements
Sjögren disease	↓ collections	↑ collections	
Thrombophlebitis	↑	↑	+ vessel wall
Thrombosis	↑	↑	– central
Tuberculoma	↓ →	↑ centrally	+ total lesion or capsule

↓   = hypointense
→   = isointense, sometimes with reference to a structure of similar intensity
↑   = hyperintense
CSF = cerebrospinal fluid

Temporal Bone

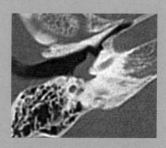

2 Radiologic Anatomy of the Temporal Bone

Today, computed tomography (CT) is the most frequently used tool to evaluate the temporal bone. It is used not only to detect pathology, but also as an evaluation tool preoperatively and during operative procedures. Preoperatively, CT may be helpful in decisions about the most optimal surgical approach and may help minimize complications during surgery.

Magnetic resonance imaging (MRI) is used for detecting retrocochlear pathology and intracranial pathology, although it may have a complementary value in evaluating the patency and fluid contents of the inner ear structures. Radiologic anatomy with regard to MRI will be discussed in Chapter 4.

Plain films of the skull to evaluate the temporal bone consist of projections described by Schüller and Stenvers. These projections have been used as a screening tool, but are no longer considered very useful. The Stenvers projection is useful after cochlear implantation to evaluate the position of the electrode in case of difficult insertion (see **Fig. 2.1**). In trauma cases, plain films give an impression of the integrity of the system, but this is usually evaluated with CT.

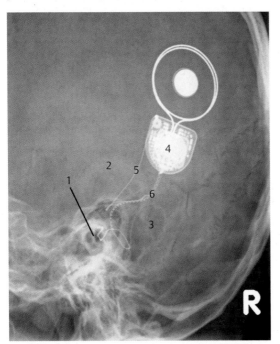

Fig. 2.1 Traditional Stenvers radiographic projection. This projection is currently used for, e.g., cochlear implantation to demonstrate the position of the electrode (1). In addition, the radiograph shows the cartilage of the outer ear (2), degree of pneumatization and aeration of the mastoid (3), the processor of the implant (4), the reference electrode (5), and the active electrode (6).

Evaluating a CT Scan of the Temporal Bone

For a systematic and complete analysis, a CT scan of the temporal bone should be evaluated in a standardized manner. An axial evaluation is best started by using cranial slices consisting of only a few structures that can be recognized more easily, to more caudal slices with a somewhat more complex anatomy. Coronal evaluation is best started anteriorly with recognition of the mandibular structures, followed by evaluation of the more posterior slices.

A comprehensive list of evaluation points is given below. In practice, documentation of the findings must be accurate, mentioning not only pathological findings but also the state of essential normal structures. Of course, not every point in the list below needs to be noted in the medical file.

Mastoid Region
- Presence and extension of the pneumatization.
- Contents of the mastoid cells (air, fluid, soft tissue).
- Position of sigmoid sinus.
- Appearance of the bony trabecular structures: intact, destruction.
- Aspect of the lateral bony border of the mastoid.
- Aspect of the bony borders of the posterior and middle fossa.
- Position and integrity of the vertical part of facial nerve canal.

Middle Ear
- Contents: loss of aeration.
- Localization and aspect of masses.
- Ossicular chain: dislocation, destruction, ankylosis.
- Appearance of the round and oval window niche.
- Aspect of the horizontal part of the facial nerve canal.
- Aspect of the region of the geniculate ganglion.
- Aspect of the ear drum: thickened, retracted.
- Position and aspect of the carotid artery, bony coverage.
- Position and aspect of the jugular bulb, bony coverage.

Inner Ear and the Petrous Apex
- Cochlea: demineralization of bony capsule, presence of the modiolus, aspect of cochlear windings and the cochlear lumen, ossification.
- Appearance of vestibular parts and semicircular canals, intact borders, ossification.
- Aspect of the internal auditory meatus: widened, irregular bony destruction, narrowed.
- Pathway of the facial nerve to the geniculate ganglion.

- Aspect of vestibular and cochlear aqueduct.
- Aspect of the petrous apex: spongy or pneumatized, secretions, smooth or irregular masses.

External Auditory Canal
- Stenosis, partial or total atresia.
- Integrity of the bony and cartilage parts.
- Exostoses and accumulation of debris.
- Extensive or irregular bony destruction.

Axial Slices through the Temporal Bone from Cranial to Caudal

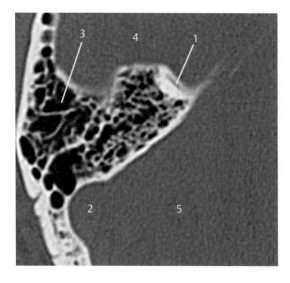

Fig. 2.2   Axial slice through the temporal bone.
1 Anterior semicircular canal
2 Sigmoid sinus
3 Highly pneumatized and aerated mastoid
4 Middle cranial fossa
5 Posterior cranial fossa

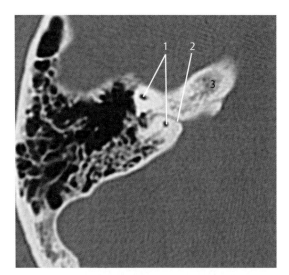

Fig. 2.3   Axial slice through the temporal bone.
1 Anterior semicircular canal
2 Subarcuate artery canal
3 Petrous apex: spongy bone or fatty marrow

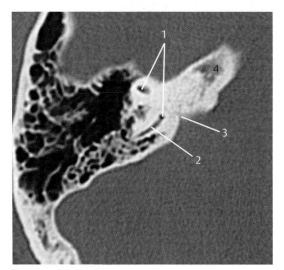

Fig. 2.4   Axial slice through the temporal bone.
1 Anterior semicircular canal
2 Posterior semicircular canal
3 Superior aspect of the internal auditory canal
4 Petrous apex (non-pneumatized)

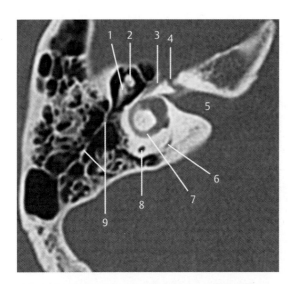

Fig. 2.5 Axial slice through the temporal bone.

1 Incus
2 Malleus head
3 Facial nerve
4 Geniculate ganglion
5 Internal auditory canal
6 Vestibular aqueduct
7 Horizontal semicircular canal
8 Posterior semicircular canal
9 Koerner septum

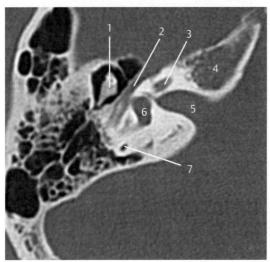

Fig. 2.6 Axial slice through the temporal bone.

1 Incus body and part of the malleus head anteriorly
2 Horizontal portion of the facial nerve
3 Basal turn of cochlea
4 Petrous apex
5 Internal auditory canal
6 Vestibule
7 Posterior semicircular canal

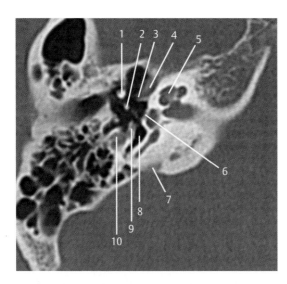

Fig. 2.7 Axial slice through the temporal bone.
1 Handle of malleus
2 Lenticular process of incus
3 Cochleariform process
4 Tensor tympani muscle
5 Cochlear modiolus
6 Footplate with stapes suprastructure
7 Vestibular aqueduct
8 Tympanic sinus
9 Pyramidal process (stapedius muscle)
10 Fusion of facial nerve and chorda tympani

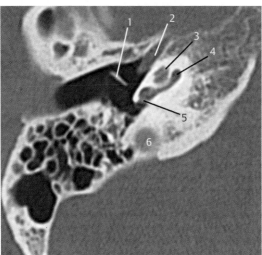

Fig. 2.8 Axial slice through the temporal bone.
1 Manubrium of malleus
2 Mucosa of eustachian tube
3 Middle and apical turns of cochlea
4 Basal turn of cochlea
5 Round window
6 Roof of jugular bulb

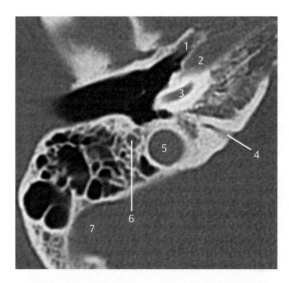

Fig. 2.9 Axial slice through the temporal bone.

1 Tympanic orifice of eustachian tube
2 Internal carotid artery
3 Basal turn of cochlea
4 Cochlear aqueduct
5 Jugular bulb
6 Vertical portion of the facial nerve
7 Sigmoid sinus

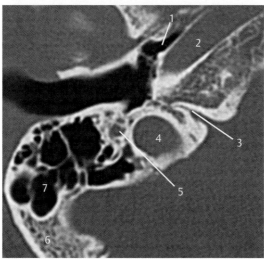

Fig. 2.10 Axial slice through the temporal bone.

1 Eustachian tube
2 Internal carotid artery
3 Cochlear aqueduct
4 Jugular bulb
5 Vertical part of facial nerve
6 Spongy bone of mastoid (no secretions)
7 Well-aerated mastoid anteriorly

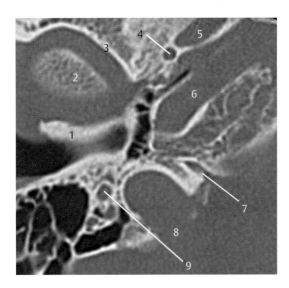

Fig. 2.11   Axial slice through the temporal bone.

1 Anterior part of the bony external auditory canal
2 Mandibular condyle
3 Anterior part of temporomandibular joint
4 Foramen spinosum
5 Foramen ovale
6 Internal carotid artery
7 Cochlear aqueduct
8 Jugular bulb
9 Facial nerve (mastoid part)

Coronal Slices through the Temporal Bone from Anterior to Posterior

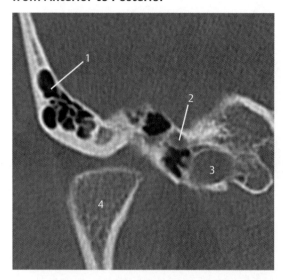

Fig. 2.12   Coronal slice through the temporal bone.
1 Well-pneumatized and aerated mastoid
2 Region of the geniculate ganglion
3 Internal carotid artery
4 Mandibular condyle

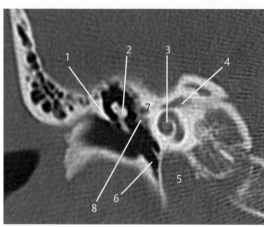

Fig. 2.13   Coronal slice through the temporal bone.
1 Scutum
2 Malleus head in epitympanic recess
3 Cochlear turns
4 Internal auditory meatus
5 Internal carotid artery
6 Anterior hypotympanum and tympanic orifice of eustachian tube
7 Horizontal part of facial nerve
8 Cochleariform process

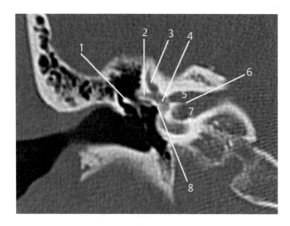

Fig. 2.14   Coronal slice through the temporal bone.

1 Long process of the incus connecting to the stapes suprastructure
2 Horizontal semicircular canal
3 Anterior semicircular canal
4 Vestibule
5 Region of facial nerve
6 Crista falciformis
7 Region of the cochlear nerve
8 Footplate in oval window niche

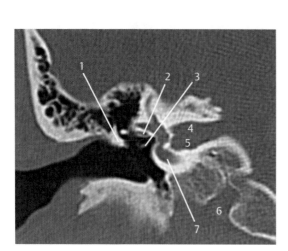

Fig. 2.15   Coronal slice through the temporal bone.

1 Scutum
2 Facial nerve
3 Stapes suprastructure
4 Region of the superior vestibular nerve
5 Region of the inferior vestibular nerve
6 Hypoglossal nerve canal
7 Basal turn of cochlea

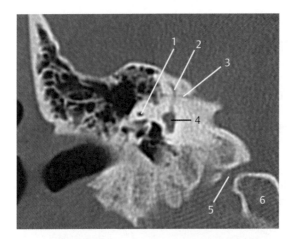

Fig. 2.16   Coronal slice through the temporal bone.
1 Horizontal semicircular canal
2 Posterior semicircular canal
3 Subarcuate artery canal
4 Vestibule
5 Petro-occipital fissure
6 Occipital condyle

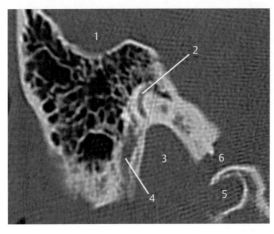

Fig. 2.17   Coronal slice through the temporal bone.
1 Bony tegmen (also seen on previous views); above this is the temporal lobe
2 Posterior semicircular canal
3 Jugular bulb
4 Vertical portion of facial nerve, with the stylomastoid foramen caudally
5 Hypoglossal canal
6 Petro-occipital fissure

3 Pathology of the Temporal Bone

Pathology of the External Auditory Canal

Inclusion Cholesteatoma and Atresia of the External Auditory Canal

Differential Diagnosis
- Any benign mass in the region of the external auditory canal, post-traumatic cholesteatoma of the external auditory canal, or cholesteatoma due to secondary stenosis of the external auditory canal as a result of chronic cicatrizing external otitis or bony stenosis due to fibrous dysplasia or exostosis in the lateral part of the external auditory canal.
- Aural atresia is often related to syndromes such as Treacher Collins, Crouzon, Nager, Goldenhar, Klippel–Feil, and Pierre Robin.

Points of Evaluation
- Expansion toward and/or destruction of the temporomandibular joint and toward the middle ear structures, abscess formation, and osteomyelitis and (intracranial) spread of infection.
- In case of aural atresia (first branchial groove anomaly), other dysmorphic features may be present too, especially in case of syndromal comorbidity.
- Particular attention needs to be paid to:
  - the appearance of the middle ear cavity and mastoid pneumatization
  - signs of ankylosis or malformation of the ossicular chain
  - presence of inner ear deformities, the round and oval windows and the vestibular aqueduct
  - aberrations in the anterior and/or lateral course of the facial nerve, which may complicate surgery.

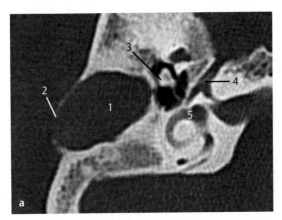

Fig. 3.1 a–c Patient with Treacher Collins syndrome and purulent discharge from a pinpoint external auditory canal.

a CT, axial. Expanding, round, smooth-bordered lesion (1) in the cranial part of the mastoid with partial destruction of the cortex (2). The head of the malleus is possibly dysmorphic and ankylotic (3). Note the geniculate ganglion (4) with a clearly visible greater petrosal nerve canal anteriorly. The vestibule and horizontal semicircular canal (5) are normal.

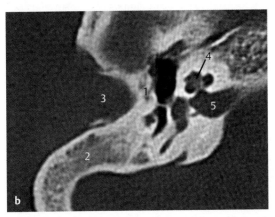

b CT, axial. More caudally, osseous atresia of the external auditory canal is observed with osseous occlusion (1). The mastoid is not pneumatized (2). Lateral to the atresia is an expanding mass (3), suggestive of inclusion cholesteatoma, filling the meatus. The cochlea (4) and internal auditory canal (5) show normal features.

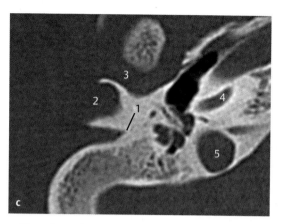

Fig. 3.1c

c CT, axial. On a lower slice, a narrowed and endingobstructed meatus is observed (1), as well as an expansile mass (2) near the temporomandibular joint (3) without signs of destruction. The slice is taken at the level of the basal cochlear turn (4) and of the roof a high jugular bulb (5).

Exostoses of the External Auditory Canal

Differential Diagnosis

- Exostoses are frequently multiple and bilateral.
- An osteoma of the external auditory canal is most often unilateral, isolated, and round in shape.
- Fibrous dysplasia has a specific appearance on computed tomography (CT) and typically is not limited to the external auditory canal (see also "Fibrous Dysplasia" [1] and [2]).
- Clinically, exostoses can be easily differentiated from soft-tissue tumors by palpation.

Points of Evaluation

- In patients with aural discharge, chronic otitis may be the result of infected epithelial stasis.
- In cases with a narrowed orifice and meatus, a meatoplasty might be considered for better aeration and cleaning options. Furthermore, CT might be reassuring, showing a normal aerated middle ear.

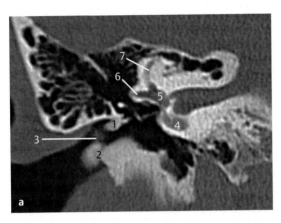

Fig. 3.2 a   Patient referred by his general practitioner because of abnormalities in the outer ear canal.

a CT, axial. Small exostoses are visualized in the roof of the external auditory canal near the annulus (1), and a larger one laterally on the floor of the meatus (2). Although some accumulation of cerumen (3) is present, hearing did not seem to be compromised, and there was no discharge. Also clearly seen are the basal cochlear turn (4), vestibule (5), and horizontal (6) and anterior (7) semicircular canals.

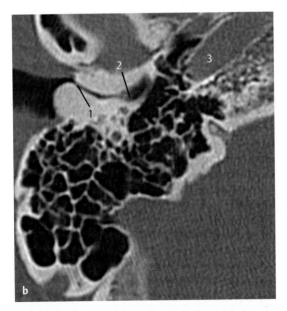

Fig. 3.2 b   Another patient with more extensive exostoses.

b CT, axial. Only a small lumen remains (1), with accumulation of cerumen or epithelium more medially (2) with a high risk of impaction and development of an inclusion cholesteatoma. Note the internal carotid artery (3), indicating the caudal orientation of this slice.

Stenosis of the External Auditory Canal

Differential Diagnosis

- Clinically, the fibrous wall has a classic appearance with a smooth and dry cicatrized skin surface. In patients with active mucosal proliferation, malignant external otitis must be considered.
- Secondary stenosis might be due to trauma (see "Skull Base Fractures") or previous canal surgery with cicatrization of the external auditory canal.
- Expanding lesions might indicate soft-tissue tumors such as (secondary) cholesteatoma, ceruminous gland tumors, and squamous cell carcinomas.

Points of Evaluation

- Beware of accumulation of cerumen or epithelium behind the fibrous wall, and exclude deeper pathology in the middle ear. In most cases, the fibrous wall can be surgically separated from the inner layers of the eardrum without opening the middle ear.
- In cases of malignant external otitis or secondary cholesteatoma, deeper pathologies (e.g., to the facial nerve) are of special interest.

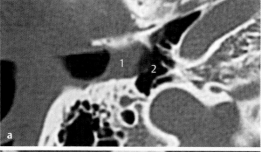
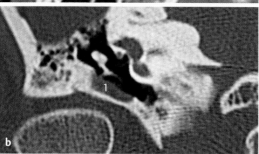

Fig. 3.3 a, b Patient with a history of chronic otitis externa.
a CT, axial. Chronic external otitis may lead to cicatrizing fibrous changes in the wall (1) of the external auditory canal. In this patient, the fibrous wall is located on the external side of the eardrum, resulting in conductive hearing loss. The middle ear is normal (2), excluding additional pathology.
b CT, coronal. The fibrous wall (1) seen in **Fig. 3.3 a** is also seen on this anteriorly located coronal slice. The pathology on this view is limited laterally by the malleus and the eardrum.

Malignant External Otitis or Necrotizing External Otitis

Differential Diagnosis

Malignant masses such as ceruminous gland tumors, basal cell tumors, and squamous cell tumors with destructive characteristics, and growth of tumors from regional areas.

Points of Evaluation

- Risk of facial nerve damage, which may lead to paresis or paralysis, as a result of extensive destruction of the area of the facial nerve, although bacterial spread may precede the signs of bony destruction.
- Beware of deeper pathologies, such as middle ear infection or intracranial complications, and risk factors such as diabetes. A swab may reveal *Pseudomonas aeruginosa* in most patients, or *Aspergillus* species in human immunodeficiency virus (HIV)-positive patients.
- Malignant masses can present with the same destructive growth pattern as malignant external otitis.

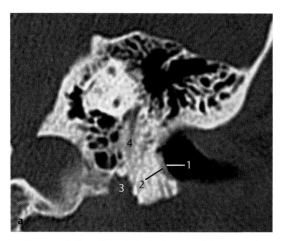

Fig. 3.4 a Patient with severe auricular pain and some discharge.

a CT, coronal. Necrotizing lesion in the floor of the external auditory canal (1). Clinically, erosive bone lesions (2) with purulent debris and denuded bone were evident. Spread of infection to the facial nerve at the point where it exits the stylomastoid foramen (3), or in its vertical portion (4), is a serious risk and complication.

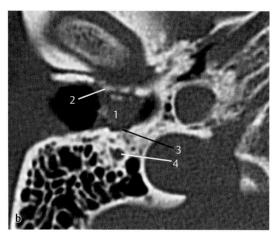

Fig. 3.4 b Patient presenting with facial paresis.

b CT, axial. An axial slice through the debris (1) in the floor of the external auditory canal. Erosive destruction of the anterior wall (2) of the temporomandibular joint is also seen, as well as posterior bony erosion (3) extending to the facial nerve canal (4), which was involved as demonstrated clinically.

Malignancy of the External Auditory Canal—Squamous Cell Carcinoma

Differential Diagnosis

- Any regional structure that might show malignant changes, such as tumors of the external auditory canal and external ear (i.e., ceruminous gland tumors or squamous cell tumors, middle ear tumors, extended parotid gland tumors).
- Intracranial tumors rarely invade bone and frequently give rise to raised intracranial pressure with resulting symptoms.

Points of Evaluation

- Extension of bony destruction and features suggestive of infiltrative growth are associated with high morbidity, such as dysfunction of the facial nerve and inner ear.
- Adherence to vital structures, such as the internal carotid artery, may preclude surgery.
- Secondary complications, i.e., mastoiditis or otitis media, as a result of stasis of secretions due to obstruction of the eustachian tube. After radiotherapy, necrotizing osteomyelitis and mastoiditis may occur.

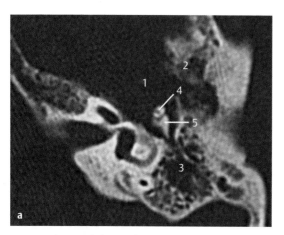

Fig. 3.5 a, b   Patient with granular proliferations in the outer ear canal.

a CT, axial. Cranial slice at the level of the horizontal canal, showing destruction of the wall of anterior epitympanum (1), irregular invasion of bone, and infiltration toward the zygomatic arch and lateral skull (2). The opacification of the mastoid (3) is probably due to secondary stasis of mucus, which in turn is caused by obstruction of the eustachian tube by the lesion. The head of malleus (4) and incus (5) are intact.

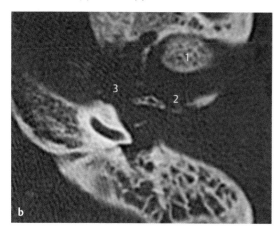

b CT, axial. Another slice at a lower level through the basal turn of the cochlea, showing anterior displacement of the mandibular condyle (1), probably due to mass effects of the tumor and extensive, irregular bony destruction in the region of the anterior external auditory canal (2), all suggestive of malignancy. In this slice, the opening of the eustachian tube (3) is obstructed by the tumor.

Pathology of the Middle Ear

Fixation of the Ossicular Chain

Differential Diagnosis
- Congenital deformities, often in relation to aural atresia (see also p. 23) and its related syndromes, such as Treacher Collins, Crouzon, Nager, Goldenhar, Klippel–Feil, and Pierre Robin.
- Fixation may also be due to otosclerosis (demineralization of the otic capsule), osteogenesis imperfecta (demineralization of otic capsule and history of multiple fractures), tympanosclerosis (myringosclerosis of the eardrum), or mass effects on the ossicular chain (congenital cholesteatoma, facial nerve schwannoma, dural prolapse, or any other middle ear tumor).
- A history of recurrent infections or trauma might be relevant.

Points of Evaluation
- As mentioned above in differential diagnosis, particular attention must be paid to patients with conductive hearing loss in combination with a normal appearing eardrum and aerated middle ear.
- In case of ankylosis of the ossicular chain, accurate evaluation of thin axial and coronal slices may reveal deformities and/or fixation.

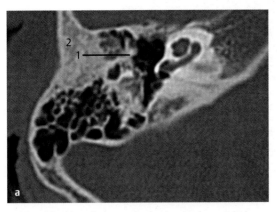

Fig. 3.6 a, b Child with congenital microtia, bony atresia of the external auditory canal, and complete conductive hearing loss.

a CT, axial. Although the conductive hearing loss might be ascribed to the atresia, the handle of the malleus (1) is fixed to the lateral bony wall of the middle ear (2), at the expected location of the atretic external auditory canal.

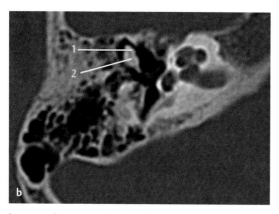

Fig. 3.6 b   Same patient as in Fig. 3.6 a.

b CT, axial. On a more superior slice through the epitympanum, the incudomalleal joint between the head of malleus (1) and the body of incus (2) is not clearly visible. These ossicles are deformed and appear as one bony mass due to fixation. No inner ear deformities are seen.

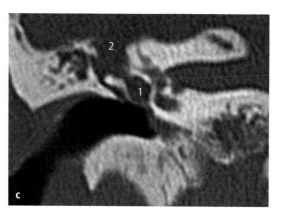

Fig. 3.6 c   In another patient with conductive hearing loss and signs of otitis media with effusion, a completely different pathology resulted in ossicular chain fixation.

c CT, coronal. Paracentesis revealed a constant loss of watery fluid, which proved to be cerebrospinal fluid. The conductive hearing loss persisted. On CT, the middle ear is fully opacified (1). The bony outline to the fossa media (tegmen tympani) was destroyed (2). At surgery, this situation was revealed to be dural prolapse with compression of the ossicular chain.

Luxation of the Ossicular Chain

Differential Diagnosis

- Congenital anomaly of the ossicular chain with a fibrous connection between the incus and stapes.
- Skull base fracture lines through the petrosal bone and opacification of the middle ear and mastoid cells due to hematoma.
- Middle ear masses with destruction of the ossicular chain, most frequently cholesteatoma (see also "Fixation of the Ossicular Chain" above). Luxation of previously placed ossicular interposition.

Points of Evaluation

- Consider the differential diagnosis, pay attention to opacifications as well as the presence and pattern of fracture lines. Always study both axial and coronal planes for accurate evaluation.
- Slowly progressive conductive hearing loss and localized opacifications in the middle ear are indicative of erosive middle ear masses.
- In all cases of trauma, clinically attention must be paid to inner ear damage and (delayed) facial nerve dysfunction.

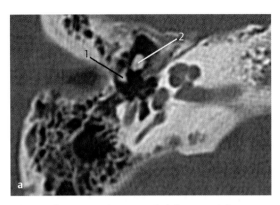

Fig. 3.7 a   Patient with aural pain and conductive hearing loss following deep cleaning of the external auditory canal with a Q-tip.

a CT, axial. Traumatic luxation with dislocation of the connection between incus (1) and malleus (2) is seen. The typical ice-cone configuration of the malleus head and incus body is lost.

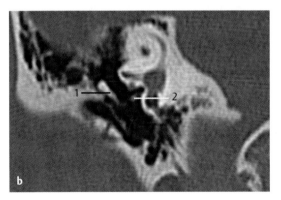

Fig. 3.7 b   This patient received a blow on the outer ear.

b CT, coronal. There was traumatic dislocation of the connection between incus (1) and stapes (2) due to barotrauma caused by sudden displacement of the eardrum. No perforation occurred, although this outcome is often seen in such patients.

Stapedectomy, Control of Piston Position

Differential Diagnosis

- Luxation of the piston due to displacement from the footplate or erosion of the incus typically presents as sudden recurrent conductive hearing loss.
- Fibrous adhesions may be found but their contribution to a renewed conductive hearing loss is doubtful.

Points of Evaluation

- Ossicular prostheses may differ as regards their degree of radiopacity and visibility on CT. For this reason fine slices are required.
- Malpositioning of the piston around the incus and possible erosions or resorption of the long process and lenticular process due to compression of the piston are difficult to evaluate on CT.

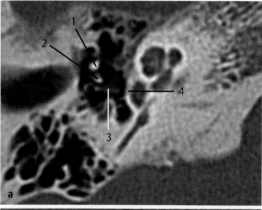

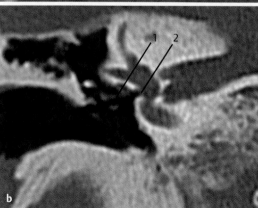

Fig. 3.8 a, b   Patient with recurrent conductive hearing loss after stapedectomy and history of reconstruction a few years earlier.

a   CT, axial. This view shows the handle of malleus (1) and posterior to it the long process of the incus (2), and a completely luxated piston (3)—from both its position in the footplate (4) and its connection to the incus.
b   CT, coronal. The dislocated prosthesis (1) outside the hole in the footplate (2). Luxation is sometimes difficult to diagnose on this view. These images emphasize the importance of combining views from different planes.

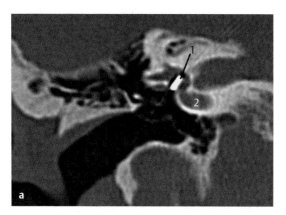

Fig. 3.9 a, b Patient with a history of bilateral stapedotomy.

a CT, coronal. The piston is positioned (1, coronal and axial) deep in the vestibule through the footplate. Note also the basal cochlear turn (2).

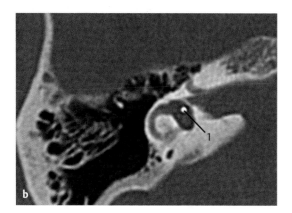

b CT, axial. Theoretically, the piston seemed to be inserted too deep into the vestibule and vestibular disorders were expected. However, this patient was operated on 30 years previously on both sides and had had no vestibular problems since.

Otosclerosis, Radiologic Signs around the Oval Niche

Differential Diagnosis

- Osteogenesis imperfecta (mostly fracture of the stapedial crus in combination with fixation of the footplate, blue sclerae depending on the genetic subtype).
- Other causes of conductive hearing loss without signs of masses in the middle ear or retraction pockets of the eardrum. See also "Fixation of the Ossicular Chain" and "Luxation of the Ossicular Chain," pages 32 and 34.

Points of Evaluation

- Absence of radiologic signs does not exclude otosclerosis.
- Early signs of otosclerotic foci on the medial wall of the cochlea are difficult to recognize, and particular attention must be paid to this situation in the evaluation of patients with conductive hearing loss of unknown cause.
- Lesions might be unilateral or bilateral.
- Family history might be positive.
- Progression of the hearing loss may occur during pregnancy.

Other radiologic signs of otosclerosis of the otic capsule are described in the inner ear section.

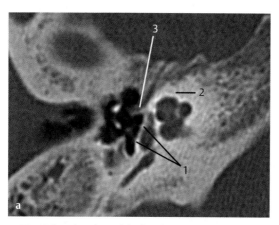

a CT, axial. At the edges of the footplate, two densities are visible (1), indicating osseous thickening, which may be considered as otosclerotic foci, especially in combination with the lucent area anterior to the footplate (more clearly demonstrated in **Fig. 3.10 b**). Slight demineralization seems to be present in the otic capsule (2). There is a good view of the cochleariform process and tensor tympani (3).

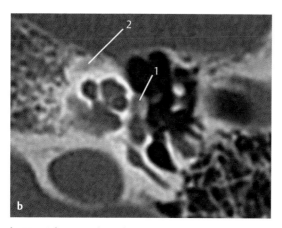

b CT, axial. Fenestral otosclerosis as illustrated by a hypodense lesion in the region of the fissula ante fenestram (1), which is frequently an early sign of otosclerosis. In most cases, the lucencies due to demineralization of the otic capsule (retrofenestral otosclerosis) are somewhat more pronounced (2); in this case this sign is very subtle or not seen.

Osteogenesis Imperfecta

Without any pathology, the stapedial crura are difficult to visualize on CT, not only due to their fine structure, but also due to the partial volume effect. This effect appears as "blurring" over sharp edges. It is due to the scanner being unable to differentiate between a small amount of high-density (e.g. crural bone) and a larger amount of lower-density (e.g. air or soft tissues) material. The processor tries to average out the two densities or structures and information is lost.

In osteogenesis imperfecta, the crura may even be thinner and more difficult to visualize, and may be more prone to fractures. Furthermore, the findings in osteogenesis imperfecta may be similar to those in otosclerosis. A more extensive case is illustrated in the section on the inner ear.

Differential Diagnosis
Otosclerosis. Other causes of conductive hearing loss without signs of masses in the middle ear or retraction pockets of the eardrum. See also "Fixation of the Ossicular Chain" and "Luxation of the Ossicular Chain," pages 32 and 34.

Points of Evaluation
In osteogenesis imperfecta affecting the middle ear, fractures of the stapedial crus are often found on middle ear inspection and/or fixation of the footplate in combination with a known (family) history of osteogenesis imperfecta. Note the typical blue sclerae of the eyes in osteogenesis imperfecta type I.

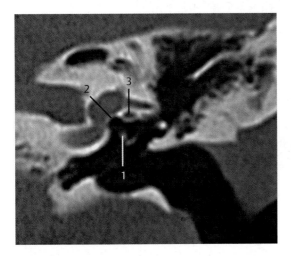

Fig. 3.11 Patient with osteogenesis imperfecta and conductive hearing loss evaluated with CT, coronal. The radiologist explicitly described an enlarged stapedial head (1). In this case, no thickening of the footplate (2) is noted. In the region of the fissula ante fenestram, a lucency as suggested on this view (3) was excluded on evaluation of sequential slices.

Gusher

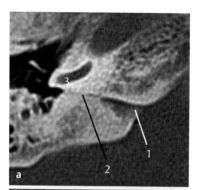

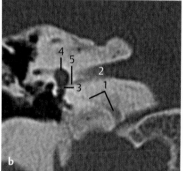

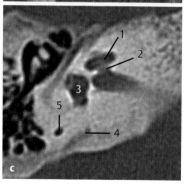

Fig. 3.12 a–c   Patient with conductive hearing loss and fixation of the footplate noted on middle ear exploration.

a CT, axial. At stapedotomy, abundant flow of inner ear fluid, the gusher phenomenon, made further surgical exploration impossible and the hole in the footplate was closed with fat and fascia of the temporal muscle. Attention must be paid to an abnormal widened cochlear aqueduct. In this case, the aperture of the cochlear aqueduct is not pathologically widened (1), although there are no agreed criteria about size in the literature. The cochlear aqueduct (2), originating from the basal cochlear turn (3), is visible on three successive 1-mm slices, suggestive of a larger size compared with non-gushers.

b CT, coronal. In the coronal slice, the cochlear aqueduct (1) is seen to run below the internal auditory canal (2) to the round window (3), and the region of the basal cochlear turn and vestibule (4). Note the inferior vestibular nerve (5). In this patient, no abnormalities were observed.

c CT, axial. Gusher is associated with other abnormal communications between the subarachnoid spaces and the perilymphatic space. Although none of these seem to be present in this patient, attention must also be paid to internal auditory canal abnormalities such as lack of a bony partition between the meatus and cochlear fundus, widened cochlear aqueduct, or cochlear anomalies (e.g., Mondini). The cochlea (1), fundus (2), vestibule (3) are normal. Also, the vestibular aqueduct (4), which according to some publications, may have a maximal diameter similar to the diameter of the posterior semicircular canal (5).

Persistent Stapedial Artery

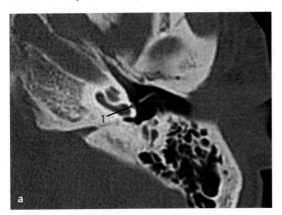

Fig. 3.13 a–d   A patient operated on for suspected otosclerosis. The surgeon encountered a surprise at the time of middle ear exploration. A pulsatile vessel was seen on the promontory, partially covered by bone, which can be suggestive of an atypical glomus tympanicum.

a CT, axial. A retrospective close examination of the CT scan revealed the stapedial artery passing along the wall of the promontory (1), between the crura of the stapes, and entering the tympanic segment of the facial canal, resulting in a broadened facial canal on CT (not shown on this slice).

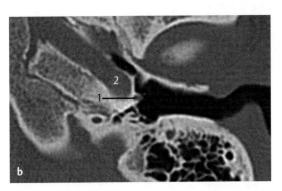

b CT, axial. The artery (1) represents the intratympanic origin of the middle meningeal artery from the internal carotid artery (2), and leaves the facial canal at the geniculate ganglion to exit the middle cranial fossa.

Fig. 3.13 c, d

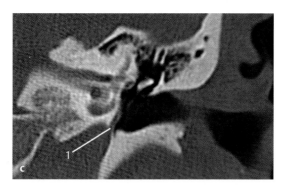

c CT, coronal. On the coronal view, its origin from the internal carotid artery and passage to the promontory is shown.

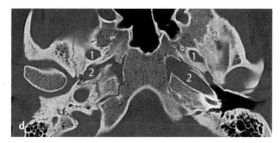

d CT, axial. On this axial skull base view, the typical absence of the foramen spinosum through which the artery usually runs, is indicative of this finding. Posteriorly, from the foramen ovale (1) and, anteriorly, from the internal carotid artery (2), the foramen spinosum should be present in normal cases (see also Chapter 4). In this case, the foramen spinosum was absent on both sides with a bilateral persistent stapedial artery. It is also known to be associated with an aberrant or aneurysmal internal carotid artery.

Glomus Tympanicum (Paraganglioma)

Differential Diagnosis
- Glomus jugulotympanicum. Endolymphatic sac tumor with destructive growth toward the middle ear (strongly associated with Von Hippel–Lindau disease; see also "Pathology of the Facial Nerve," p. 66, and Chapter 5).
- Less likely in this patient, due to the lack of evident pulsating red masses, the following must also be considered: adenoma of the middle ear and congenital cholesteatoma with a red appearance due to granulation mucositis posterior to the eardrum.

Points of Evaluation
- Glomus tympanicum is limited to the middle ear, whereas in glomus jugulotympanicum there are signs of bony destruction in the region of the jugular bulb and jugular foramen, and a salt and pepper configuration on MRI.
- Glomus jugulotympanicum is associated with higher morbidity and a less favorable outcome due to palsies of cranial nerves IX, X, and XI, and extension into structures of the neck and skull base (see also Chapter 5).

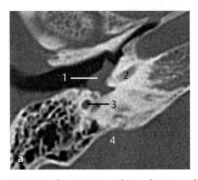 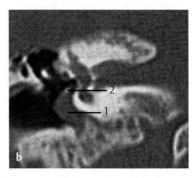

Fig. 3.14 a, b Patient with a pulsating red-blue mass posterior and caudal to the eardrum.

a CT, axial. On this axial slice at the level of the hypotympanum, a smooth-bordered lesion (1) is seen, without any destruction of the cochlea (2) or vertical part of the facial nerve canal (3). Since there seems to be no connection to the jugular bulb or jugular vein (4), this lesion may be considered to be a glomus temporale type A.

b CT, coronal. Coronal view with the hypotympanic glomus (1). The bony structures inferiorly seem intact. This patient had pulsatile tinnitus, which can be explained by the tumor being in contact with the stapedial suprastructure (2).

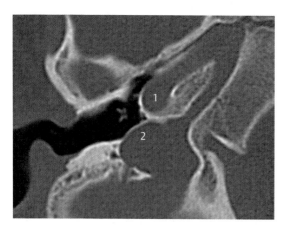

Fig. 3.15 Beware of normal anatomic variations.

CT, axial. In addition to patients with glomus tympanicum, in whom a pulsating red mass is clearly visible behind the eardrum, one must be aware of other possibilities. This figure clearly shows the danger of insertion of a tympanostomy tube (visible in the eardrum) by showing its relation and distance to the carotid artery (1) and jugular bulb (2). In case of retraction of the eardrum and/or denuded vessel or aberrant vessel course, puncturing of these vessels is a high risk and serious complication. Pathology of these vessels may be recognized by a red mass, sometimes indicating a (aberrant) carotid artery, or a dark-blue mass, indicating a high jugular bulb.

Cholesteatoma of the Middle Ear

Differential Diagnosis
Otitis media, glomus tympanicum, adenoma, adenocarcinoma, rhabdomyosarcoma, Langerhans cell histiocytosis.

Points of Evaluation
- The clinical appearance of cholesteatoma consists of a white mass behind the eardrum. Most relevant is the presence of retractions in the classic Shrapnell region or in the posterosuperior part of the eardrum toward the aditus ad antrum. Signal polyps or granulating mucositis due to infection of the contents of the pocket may mimic the presence and appearance of cholesteatoma.
- Differentiation between cholesteatoma and coexisting secretions of chronic otitis media is difficult on CT, but MRI with diffusion-weighted imaging (DWI) can assist in this (see also "Pathology of the Mastoid," page 48, and Chapter 5).

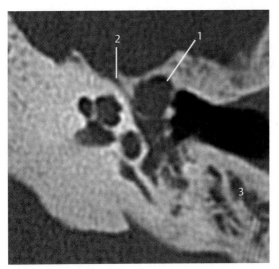

Fig. 3.16 Patient with periodic puralent discharge and hearing loss.

CT, axial. The most frequently encountered mass in the middle ear is cholesteatoma, and therefore it is (also) shown in this chapter. In this patient, there is complete opacification of the middle ear by a smooth-bordered soft-tissue mass with bony erosions in the anterior part of the middle ear (1). In this case, not only was the epitympanum filled with cholesteatoma, but also the region of the eustachian tube (2) with obstruction and stasis of secretions in the mastoid (3). Differentiation between cholesteatoma and secretions is not possible on CT.

Adenoma of the Middle Ear

Differential Diagnosis

Cholesteatoma with or without otitis media, adenocarcinoma (more infiltrating characteristics), glomus tympanicum, rhabdomyosarcoma, Langerhans cell histiocytosis.

Points of Evaluation

Evaluation of extension to critical structures such as the internal carotid artery and facial nerve is essential when considering whether complete surgical removal is possible.

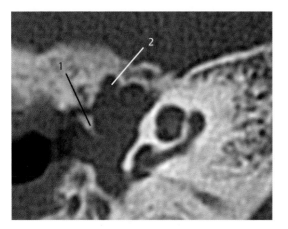

Fig. 3.17 Patient with slowly progressive loss without discharge from the ear.

CT, axial. Expansive lesion with lytic destruction of the malleus and incus (1, not clearly shown on this view) as well as anterior bony destruction (2), which seems to be smooth bordered (non-infiltrative). However, at surgical exploration, a glassy granular mass with infiltrative characteristics was found.

Pathology of the Mastoid

Cholesteatoma

Differential Diagnosis
Benign tumors with expansive characteristics but without infiltration of the surrounding bone. Otitis and mastoiditis may coexist.

Points of Evaluation
- On coronal slices, particular attention must be paid to the scutum, which might be partially eroded in cases of retraction pockets or cholesteatoma. The ossicular chain might be slightly eroded, especially the long process and lenticular process of the incus, as well as the stapes head.
- Compression of the facial nerve or destruction of the semicircular canals must be evaluated, as well as the bony outline of the posterior cranial fossa and middle cranial fossa (tegmen). An MRI will be complementary in suspected intracranial extension.

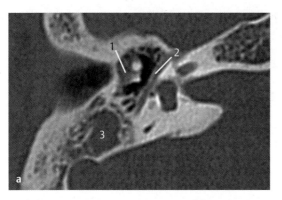

Fig. 3.18 a–c Patient with a Shrapnell retraction pocket.

a CT, axial. There is localized opacification on the lateral side of the malleus and incus (1) at the level of the facial nerve (2), suggestive of a soft-tissue mass. Opacification of the mastoid antrum (3), with a smooth-bordered expansile appearance and destruction of bony trabeculae, are more suggestive of cholesteatoma than mucous secretions.

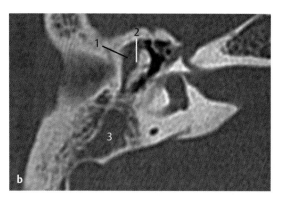

Fig. 3.18 b, c

b CT, axial. On a higher slice at the level of the malleus head and body of the incus, the opacification (1) persists and seems to result in slight lateral erosion of the ossicular chain (2). Note the persistent opacification of the mastoid (3), probably due to coexisting accumulation of serous or purulent secretions.

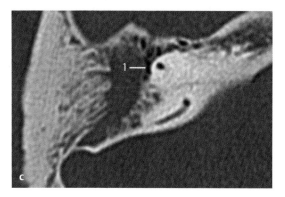

c CT, axial. More cranially in the epitympanum, a connection to the posterior mastoid is demonstrated. There is also an expansive appearance anteriorly (1), which seems to consist of a mass going through the aditus ad antrum to the mastoid with loss of bony trabeculae. In combination with the Shrapnell pocket, these images are consistent with a cholesteatoma.

Labyrinthine Fistula due to Cholesteatoma

Differential Diagnosis
- All other benign tumors with expansive characteristics from the middle ear and mastoid.
- Less frequently and with a typical location and growth pattern (see separate sections): endolymphatic sac tumor and glomus jugulotympanicum.

Points of Evaluation
- Bony dehiscences of the horizontal part of the facial nerve canal on CT may be due to a partial volume effect or may be a normal congenital finding in a minority of patients.
- Pneumatic otoscopy or manipulation of the outer ear may evoke vertigo by mechanical stimulation of the vestibular fluid contents, the so-called fistula symptom.
- At surgery, there is a greater risk of deafness but in most cases the matrix of the cholesteatoma can be dissected from the inner ear compartments without causing the leakage of inner ear fluids, thus preventing hearing loss. Intracranial complications may arise from infected cholesteatoma (see also Chapter 5).

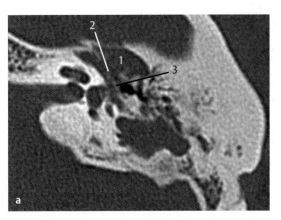

Fig. 3.19 a–c Patient with vertigo attacks, particularly on manipulation of the outer ear, indicative of the fistula symptom.

a CT, axial. Note the smooth-bordered opacification suggestive of cholesteatoma in the anterior part of the middle ear (1), at the level of the facial nerve; there may be bone dehiscence in the anterior part of the facial nerve (2), while the bony shell is still visible in the posterior part (3).

Fig. 3.19 b, c

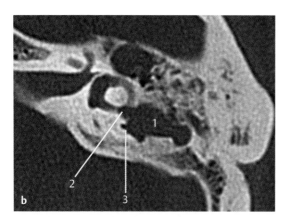

b CT, axial. In this slice through the horizontal semicircular canal, the opacification in the mastoid (1), suggestive of a mass of cholesteatoma, protrudes into the posterior part of the horizontal canal (2). Also, there is local bone destruction of the posterior semicircular canal (3).

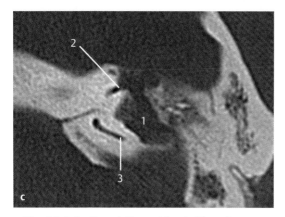

c CT, axial. A slice through the cranial part of the epitympanum shows complete opacification due to the mass (1). At the anterior part of the anterior semicircular canal (2), a third bony dehiscence is observed. At this slice, the cranial part of the posterior canal is intact (3).

In conclusion, in this patient, all three semicircular canals demonstrated fistulae due to bony destruction by the cholesteatoma.

Congenital Cholesteatoma

Differential Diagnosis

- Adenoma of the middle ear. Endolymphatic sac tumor originates in the region of the vestibular aqueduct and may grow caudally toward the jugular bulb, and also toward the infralabyrinthine region. An endolymphatic sac tumor is more destructive and infiltrative with extensions to the middle cranial fossa.
- Schwannoma and metastasis are less likely.

Points of Evaluation

- Invasion of the inner ear structures and internal auditory canal, which might complicate surgery. Adherence to the jugular bulb and facial nerve.
- Most congenital cholesteatomas or epidermoids are encountered in the petrosal apex or cerebellopontine angle (see also Chapter 5).

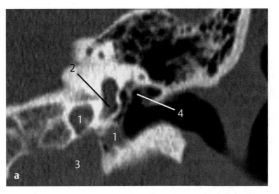

Fig. 3.20 a–c Patient with a Shrapnell pocket that was quite suggestive of cholesteatoma on clinical examination.

a CT, coronal. CT excluded deeper invagination, but revealed other pathology. Coincidentally, an expansive infralabyrinthine opacification (1) is demonstrated on this slice through the vestibule and the start of the basal cochlear turn (2). The mass is located superiorly to the jugular bulb (3), which demonstrates an intact bony covering. Furthermore, a small Shrapnell pocket is seen (4), which was neither correlated nor connected to the mass at surgical exploration.

Fig. 3.20 b, c

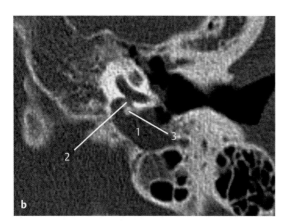

b CT, axial. On this axial infralabyrinthine slice, the position of the mass (1) is posterior to the cochlea, without any component in the middle ear, suggestive of congenital cholesteatoma. Note the expansion and bony destruction toward the fundus of the cochlea (2). The white dot (3) is suggestive of a sequestered bone fragment, which was confirmed at surgical exploration.

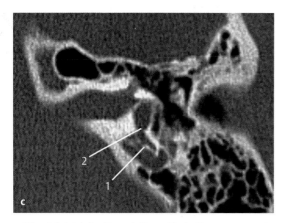

c CT, axial. Axial slice through the vestibule. The mass seems to be invading the posterior semicircular canal (1) near its connection to the vestibule (2). This congenital cholesteatoma was surgically removed with confirmation of several fistulae to the inner ear structures but with preservation of inner ear function.

Skull Base Fractures

Differential Diagnosis
- When there is clinical suspicion of a fracture, systematic evaluation of the CT scan is necessary, preferably on thin sections through the skull base.
- The difference between longitudinal and transverse fractures is not clinically relevant.
- Suture lines or bony vascular canals, so-called pseudofractures, may be misinterpreted as skull base fractures.

Points of Evaluation
- Hearing loss and vertigo are suggestive of fractures through inner ear structures (mainly transverse fractures) or conductive hearing loss due to luxation of the ossicular chain (mainly longitudinal fractures), and hematoma of the middle ear. Leakage of cerebrospinal fluid may be persistent and carries a risk of infection; therefore the patient may need surgical closure. Beware of epidural hematoma secondary to disruption of the middle meningeal artery. The anterior bony wall of the external auditory canal must be inspected to look for the impression of the mandibular condyle caused by the trauma.
- At the time of trauma, before a sedative or anesthetic is administered, facial nerve evaluation is critical to determine the presence of acute and complete paralysis. In these cases, the course of the facial nerve on CT must be evaluated carefully for presence of dislocations or bone fragments which may need surgical exploration. Delayed facial nerve dysfunction may occur from edema at a later stage and may be managed conservatively.

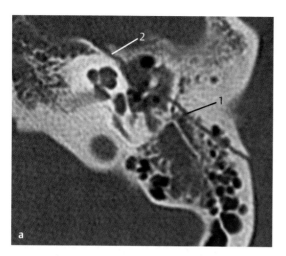

Fig. 3.21 a, b   Skull base fractures after head trauma.

a CT, axial. Patient with head trauma showing a fracture line through the mastoid (1) extending just anterior to the cochlea (2). Luxation of the ossicular chain might be expected in this case. Opacification of the mastoid and middle ear is most often due to hematoma. The fracture line in the length of the temporal bone is seen most frequently, and is a so-called **longitudinal fracture**.

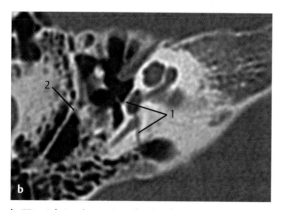

b CT, axial. Another patient after head trauma with leakage of cerebrospinal fluid and immediate facial nerve paralysis showing a fracture line through the vestibule posteriorly and the footplate (1), mostly likely due to damage at the first genu of the facial nerve. The ossicular chain seems to be intact. Note the nicely formed Koerner septum (2). A fracture perpendicular to the axis of the temporal bone is a so-called **transverse fracture**.

Malformations, Treacher Collins

Differential Diagnosis
Aural atresia and middle ear deformities are often related to syndromes such as Treacher Collins, Crouzon, Nager, Goldenhar, Klippel–Feil, and Pierre Robin.

Points of Evaluation
In deformities of the temporal bone, pay particular attention to the:
- External auditory canal, bony or fibrous atresia, appearance and position of the mandibular condyle and temporomandibular joint.
- Appearance of the middle ear cavity and mastoid pneumatization.
- Signs of ankylosis or disconnections of the ossicular chain.
- Presence of inner ear deformities, the round and oval windows, and the vestibular aqueduct.
- Aberrations in the course and anterior displacement of the facial nerve, which may complicate surgery.

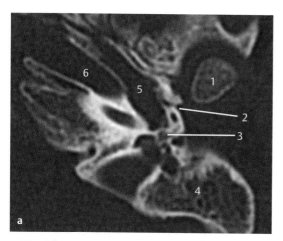

Fig. 3.22 a, b Patient with Treacher Collins syndrome and complete conductive hearing loss.

a CT, axial. For orientation, this is a slice through the basal cochlear turn and the mandibular condyle (1). Behind the condyle, the bony part of the external auditory canal is absent in combination with atresia of the external auditory canal in which the medial part demonstrates complete bony closure (2). The facial nerve (3) is immediately behind this, carrying a risk for damage at surgical exploration, especially because the mastoid is not pneumatized (4). The middle ear (5), lateral to the internal carotid artery (6), is not aerated and looks merely like an enlarged eustachian tube.

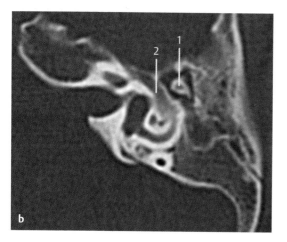

b CT, axial. On a more cranial slice, a small nonaerated epitympanic space can be recognized, containing a fused and dysmorphic malleus head and incus body (1). There is no pneumatization of the mastoid. The facial nerve is shortened in its passage through the middle ear (2). In this case, inner ear structures had a normal appearance.

Fibrous Dysplasia (1)

Differential Diagnosis
Localized to the dural outlines, these finding might also be suggestive of:
- Meningioma (see also Chapter 5).
- Paget disease (initial involvement of marrow-containing periosteal bone).
- Osteopetrosis (diffuse bony sclerosis without the increased volume of bone see in fibrous dysplasia).
- Extreme forms of otosclerosis (limited to the otic capsule).
- Osteogenesis imperfecta.
- Radionecrosis.

Points of Evaluation
- Radiologically on CT, enlargement of bone with intact cortical outlines and a dense "ground glass" appearance is characteristic of fibrous dysplasia. Fibrous dysplasia incidentally found on MRI may be confused with a malignancy.
- In meningioma, bony outlines can be irregular and signs of hyperostosis can be found as well as a dural tail. Sometimes intracranial calcifications might be indicative of an intracranial meningioma.
- In progressive disease, there is encroachment of neural structures and foramina in the skull base, with resultant neurologic and vascular deficits. The external auditory canal may be narrowed and medial to the stenosis; an inclusion cholesteatoma might develop.
- Surgical procedures are limited to prevent complications of encroachment of critical structures and treatment of chronic infections in the middle ear cavity. In obstruction of the auditory canal, extra attention must be paid to the potential risk of inclusion cholesteatoma.

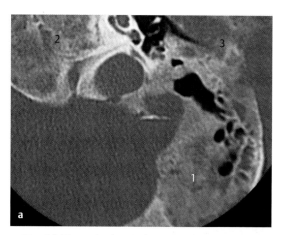

a CT, axial. Fibrous dysplasia is characterized by replacement of medullary bone by abnormally proliferating fibrous tissue, resulting in asymmetric distortion and expansion of bone. It may be restricted to a single osseous structure (monostotic fibrous dysplasia) or involve multiple bones (polyostotic fibrous dysplasia). In this patient, a polyostotic variant shows extensive distortions of the mastoid (1), petrosal apex (2), and anterior skull base (3). In the region of the temporomandibular joint, functional disorders of the temporomandibular joints and stenosis of the external auditory canal may develop.

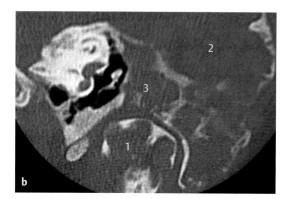

b CT, coronal. The mandibular condyle (1) is hardly recognizable as such, and bony outlines of the middle cranial fossa are barely visible (2) with the risk of damage in surgical explorations. The region of the external auditory canal is completely obstructed (3).

Iatrogenic Fenestration

Differential Diagnosis
- A noniatrogenic fistula of the horizontal canal must be considered, especially in cases where there is no known history of fenestration.
- Cholesteatoma, or other compressing tumors, resulting in a labyrinthine fistula, may have been removed during previous surgery.

Points of Evaluation
- In fenestrated patients, no actual compression due to masses will be seen.
- Beware of suction of the cavity for cleaning. This must be performed very carefully to prevent severe vertigo and inner ear dysfunction.

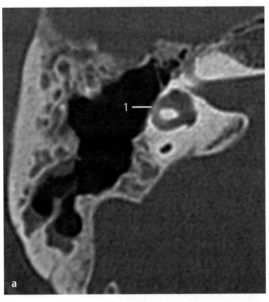

Fig. 3.24a, b History of hearing loss and unknown surgical intervention many years before.

a CT, axial. Before the availability of microsurgical techniques and the use of ossicular replacement prostheses, mobilization of the footplate was carried out in patients with otosclerosis to restore hearing. An alternative procedure, as shown in this figure, was iatrogenic fenestration of the horizontal semicircular canal (1) in combination with a modified radical cavity, in which sound is directly transmitted to the inner ear structures.

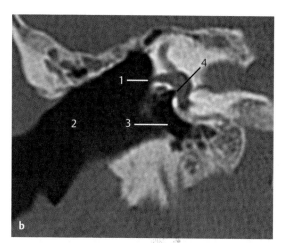

Fig. 3.24 b

b CT, coronal. On a coronal view, the fenestration (1) is in direct contact with the enlarged external auditory canal (2). A small remnant of the middle ear is visible (3), without ossicular reconstruction on the footplate (4).

Modified Radical Cavity, Persistent Infections

Differential Diagnosis
- Underlying or additional pathologies: inclusion or residual cholesteatoma, eustachian tube dysfunction, residual mastoid cells, insufficient cleaning of the cavity, mucosal overgrowth and resulting bacterial or fungal infections.
- An insufficiently enlarged entrance to the external auditory canal might exacerbate pathology in a (modified) radical cavity due to insufficient aeration and inability to clean the cavity.

Points of Evaluation
- Attention must be paid to the above-mentioned presence of residual cells. Residual cholesteatoma may present as smooth-bordered, rounded swellings covered by an epithelial or mucosal lining. In cases of destruction of the bony outline to the middle of posterior cranial fossa, a complementary MRI might be helpful for evaluating the extent of the pathology and its relation to intracranial structures.
- DWI is especially helpful in discriminating between recurrent or residual cholesteatoma and granulation tissue.

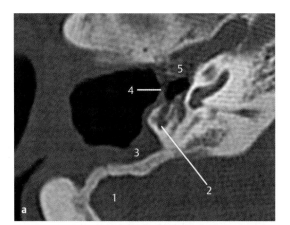

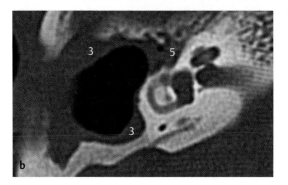

Fig. 3.25 a, b Persistent secretion from a modified radical cavity.

CT, axial. This may necessitate CT to evaluate any residual pathology. In these axial slices at the level of the cochlea and horizontal canal, no remaining mastoid cells are present, shown by the bony outline along the sigmoid sinus (1); the only remaining cell contains the facial nerve (2). Chronic mucositis is illustrated by a thickened mucosal outline (3) along the bony borders without any sign of residual mastoid cells or an underlying pathology such as cholesteatoma. Medial to the thickened eardrum (4), the middle ear is partly aerated with mucosal swelling at the orifice of the eustachian tube (5).

Osteoradionecrosis

Differential Diagnosis
Osseous dystrophies such as fibrous dysplasia (see also separate sections) or Paget disease. Chronic osteomyelitis of the temporal bone. In earlier times, patients underwent radiotherapy to treat chronic middle ear infections.

Points of Evaluation
Stasis of secretions and infections are frequently the result of eustachian tube dysfunction due to mucosal swelling and loss of ciliary function. Chronic infections may require complete surgical removal of the affected bone and long-term antibiotic treatment.

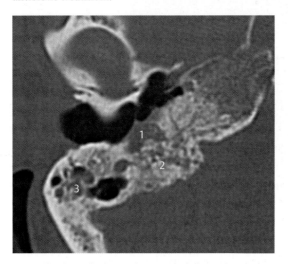

Fig. 3.26 Patient with a history of radiotherapy for a pulsating middle ear tumor.

CT, axial. After radiotherapy for a residual glomus (1), the petrosal bone has a brittle appearance with signs of bony changes, fibrosis, and necrotized areas (2). These may also develop several years after radiotherapy. Note also stasis of secretions or infection in the mastoid (3).

Dural Prolapse and Cerebrospinal Fluid Leakage

Differential Diagnosis
Schwannoma or hemangioma of the facial geniculate ganglion. Cholesteatoma or middle ear tumors with anterior expansion to the middle cranial fossa.

Points of Evaluation
Signs of infiltration or expansion. An MRI may be necessary to exclude or evaluate intracranial involvement.

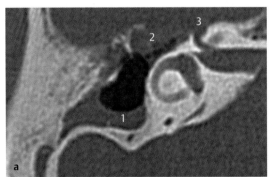

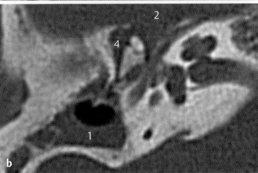

Fig. 3.27 a, b   Cerebrospinal fluid leakage after insertion of a tympanostomy tube (grommet), indicated for middle ear secretions and conductive hearing loss without any otologic history.

CT, axial. Note the residual fluid (1) on the axial CT slices. In the anterior epitympanum, opacification (2) and destruction of the bony outline to the middle fossa, possibly due to dural prolapse, is observed in the region of the geniculate ganglion (3). At surgical exploration, the bullous dural prolapse was in direct contact with the ossicular chain (4) without signs of further destruction.

Pathology of the Facial Nerve

Hemangioma of the Geniculate Ganglion

Differential Diagnosis
- Schwannoma of the facial geniculate ganglion.
- Dural prolapse from the middle fossa.
- Middle ear tumors extending anteriorly toward the middle cranial fossa.

Points of Evaluation
- Signs of infiltration or expansion. An MRI may be necessary to exclude or evaluate intracranial involvement.
- Most tumors, such as schwannoma, demonstrate more sharply defined enhancement.
- Outlines are often poorly defined in hemangiomas. A characteristic salt and pepper configuration is due to accumulation of methemoglobin and flow voids from the increased vascularization. Ossifying hemangiomas might demonstrate bone spicules.
- Hemangiomas of the facial nerve become symptomatic at an earlier stage compared with schwannomas, which might be quite large before symptoms occur.

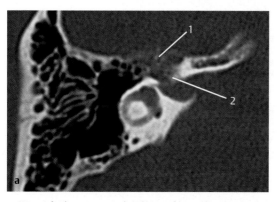

Fig. 3.28 a–c   Patient with slowly progressive, unilateral right facial nerve paresis.

a CT, axial. There is a spiculated area of bone destruction or a mass with calcifications in the region of the geniculate ganglion (1), just distal to the exit point of the facial nerve (2) from the internal auditory canal.

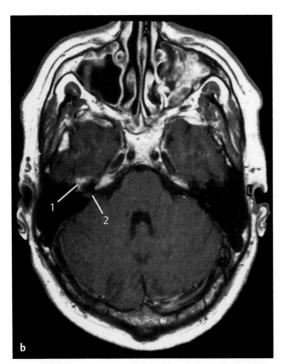

Fig. 3.28 b, c
b MRI, T1-weighted with gadolinium enhancement, axial. Contrast enhancement (1) at the location of the geniculate ganglion as demonstrated on CT. The area of enhancement is ill-defined. No enhancement is seen in the internal auditory canal (2).

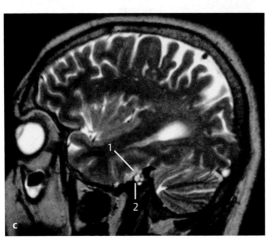

c MRI T2-weighted, sagittal. This view demonstrates the lesion anteriorly (1) from the cochlea (2). There is no sharp outline. The intensity on this T2-weighted image is suggestive of high fluid contents. Peroperatively, a friable and bloody lesion was removed, suggestive of hemangioma, which was confirmed by the pathologist.

Schwannoma of the Facial Nerve

Differential Diagnosis

In smaller schwannomas in the region of the geniculate ganglion, a hemangioma, dural prolapse from the middle fossa, or middle ear tumors with anterior expansion to the middle cranial fossa must be considered.

Points of Evaluation

- CT and MRI are complementary in the evaluation of the extension of the schwannoma to the middle or posterior cranial fossa as well as to the inner ear structures. Compared with hemangiomas, schwannomas of the facial nerve can be quite large before symptoms occur.
- Surgical removal with facial nerve grafting is only considered in (near) total paralysis of the facial nerve or when expansion of the lesion would lead to the damage of surrounding critical structures.

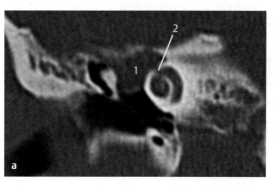

Fig. 3.29 a–c
Slowly progressive, right-sided facial nerve paresis and inner ear dysfunction.

a CT, coronal. CT demonstrates an opacification (1) in the medial and anterior epitympanum, suggestive of an expanding mass with destruction of the cochlear capsule (2) as an explanation for inner ear dysfunction.

Fig. 3.29 b, c

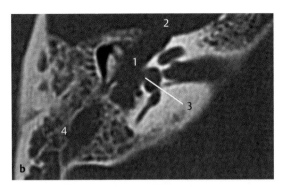

b CT, axial. Largely widened horizontal portion of the facial nerve (1) of the same patient as in **Fig. 3.29 a**, with a bony dehiscence toward the middle cranial fossa (2) and possibly extension into the vestibule (3), all signs suggesting a schwannoma of the facial nerve. Note the opacification of the mastoid (4) due to stasis of secretions as a result of eustachian tube obstruction by the schwannoma.

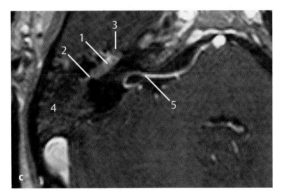

c MRI, T1-weighted with gadolinium enhancement, axial. There is a sharply defined enhancing mass suggestive of a schwannoma of the facial nerve. The anterior part of the facial nerve is enlarged (1). This is not the case in the posteriorly horizontal tympanic part of the facial nerve (2), although enhancement can also be detected in this region, suggestive of active infiltration. Protrusion or invasion into the middle cranial fossa was excluded by MRI (3). A clear difference between this schwannoma and the mastoid secretions (4), which are probably due to occlusion of the eustachian tube, is shown by the difference in signal intensity. Note the clear view of the anterior inferior cerebellar artery (5).

Endolymphatic Sac Tumor

Differential Diagnosis
Glomus jugulotympanicum, hemangioma, meningioma, middle ear tumors, chondrosarcoma, metastasis.

Points of Evaluation
- Signs of bone destruction in the region of the jugular bulb and jugular foramen.
- Cranial nerve VII–XI palsies, extension into structures of the neck and skull base (see also Chapter 5).
- An endolymphatic sac tumor has a high risk of progressive morbidity and surgical complications due to excessive bleeding and cranial nerve damage. Preoperative embolization is recommended if technically possible.
- There is a well-known higher incidence of endolymphatic sac tumor in Von Hippel–Lindau disease.

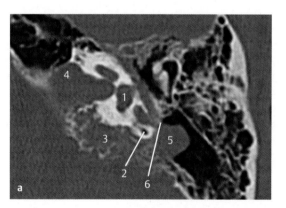

Fig. 3.30 a–c   Patient with unexplained unilateral deafness for 20 years and recent onset of progressive facial paralysis.

a CT, axial. Posterior to the vestibule (1) and posterior semicircular canal (2), an opacification of the mastoid cells with infiltrative characteristics is seen. This mass is not only confined to the region of the endolymphatic sac (3), but also shows expansive destruction of the anterior portion of the internal auditory canal (4) and extension toward the mastoid (5) and facial nerve (6).

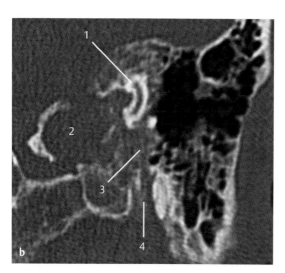

Fig. 3.30 b, c

b CT, coronal. The mass is bounded by the posterior semicircular canal (1), the jugular bulb (2) with erosion of its bony outlines, and the vertical portion of the facial nerve (3) toward the stylomastoid foramen (4).

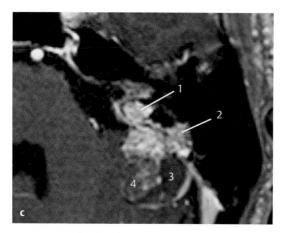

c MRI, T1-weighted with gadolinium enhancement, axial. The tumor enhances strongly with gadolinium due to its high vascularity (1). Protrusion into the mastoid (2) as seen on the CT. Note also the cystic nonenhancing components (3) and extension into the posterior cranial fossa (4).

Pathology of the Inner Ear

Malformations of the Inner Ear

Differential Diagnosis
Mondini deformity, cochlear hypoplasia, common cavity, Michel deformity.

Points of Evaluation
- Incomplete partition of the cochlea may be divided into two variants: Mondini deformity shows a normal basal cochlear turn in combination with a cystic appearance and fusion of the second and third cochlear turn, in contrast to those cases without any sign of a modiolus, scalar divisions or cribriform area. In these cases, a separate large cystic vestibule is found.
- In cases of a common cavity, only an otocystic cavity is found representing the cochlea and vestibule without further differentiation. In cases of a Michel deformity, the most severe inner ear anomaly, there is complete absence of the cochlea.

Inner ear malformations may be associated with multiple syndromes involving other organs. A multidisciplinary approach is favored to recognize this. Sometimes genetic counseling is helpful for an accurate diagnosis of syndromes.

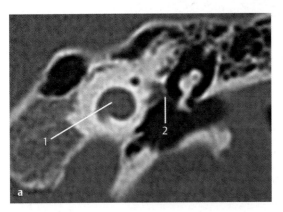

Fig. 3.31 a–c Patient with congenital deafness.

a CT, coronal. This coronal view of the cochlea does not show any bony modiolus (1). This empty cochlea is suggestive of an incomplete partition or a common cavity. Note the clear view of the cochleariform process (2).

Fig. 3.31 b, c

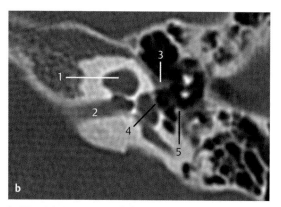

b CT, axial. Again, no modiolus or interscalar septa are visible (1). This deformity might be unilateral or bilateral. Note the clear view of a normal internal auditory canal (2), cochleariform process (3), footplate and stapes suprastructure (4), and pyramidal eminence (5).

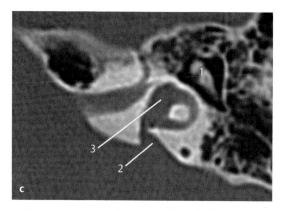

c CT, axial. Normal ossicular chain configuration (1). In Mondini deformity, deformities of the vestibular aqueduct are also present as demonstrated in this case by its shortened and enlarged appearance (2), as well as an enlarged vestibule (3). Note the normal aspect of the horizontal semicircular canal.

Malformations of the Inner Ear and Ossicular Chain

Differential Diagnosis

- Hypoplasia of the cochlea is characterized by a diminished cochlear height or shortening of the cochlea with less than 2.5 turns.
- Aplasia of one or more semicircular canals may be difficult to distinguish from labyrinthitis ossificans. Association with CHARGE, BOR, and Goldenhar syndrome has been described. Michel deformity (complete absence of the cochlea). Common cavity (only an otocystic remnant).
- Association with other syndromes involving deformities of the malleus and incus, since in most cases the embryological development of the middle and external ear is independent from the inner ear.

Points of Evaluation

This section illustrates the importance of a systematic comparison of both sides as well as the different compartments of the ear since bilateral congenital pathology may show (subtle) variations between the left and right side.

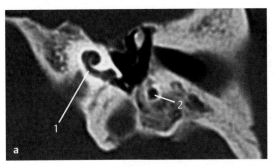

Fig. 3.32 a–c   Patient presenting with congenital mixed hearing loss.

a CT, axial. Illustrative evaluation of malformations of the inner ear as well as the middle ear. This axial slice demonstrates a cochlea consisting of only 1.5 turns (1), which might be classified a hypoplastic cochlea. Note also the nonpneumatized mastoid with the facial nerve (2).

Fig. 3.32 b, c

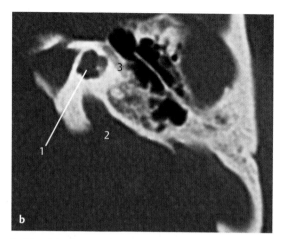

b CT, axial. This view shows an extensively enlarged vestibule with dysmorphic characteristics (1). All semicircular canals are absent, the vestibular aqueduct (2) is enlarged, and the facial nerve is normal (3).

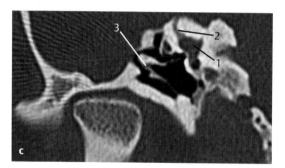

c CT, coronal. The contralateral side also shows the same enlarged vestibule (1). On this side, presence of one semicircular canal could be confirmed (2): the anterior canal. Furthermore, note the subtle underdevelopment of the ossicular chain (3).

Vestibular Aqueduct, Enlargements

Differential Diagnosis

Also related to other inner ear deformities such as Mondini, common cavity, and syndromes with otologic involvement, such as Klippel–Feil, Wildervanck, Waardenburg, Pendred, Di George, Goldenhar, and CHARGE association.

Points of Evaluation

- The width of the vestibular aqueduct may be evaluated at the midpoint of the duct in its course from its origin at the upper vestibule close to the crus commune to the aperture in the epidural space. Although lacking consensus, a midpoint width of 1.5–2 mm, or larger than twice the size of the width of the posterior semicircular canal, is considered to be pathologic. The width may also be determined and compared at its aperture in several ways, although measuring this region is complicated.
- Bilateral systematic comparison of the different parts of the inner ear, middle ear, and external ear remains essential in differentiating between normal variants and pathologic states. Knowledge of other relevant clinical symptoms is essential in syndromic cases. Genetic counseling may be helpful.

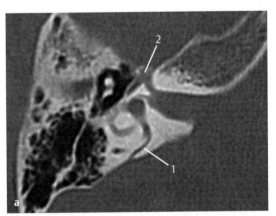

Fig. 3.33 a–c   Evaluations of size and appearance of the vestibular aqueduct.

a CT, axial. The normal vestibular aqueduct (1) in its passage from the vestibule to its junction with sinuses in the region of the sigmoid sinus. There is a clear view of the normal-appearing geniculate ganglion (2).

Fig. 3.33 b, c

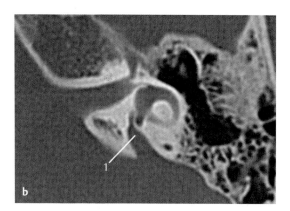

b CT, axial. In another case, a slightly enlarged vestibular aqueduct (1) is seen, which might be clinically nonsignificant.

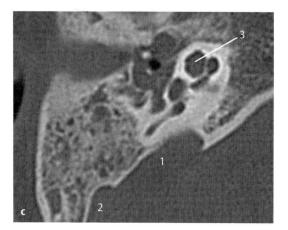

c CT, axial. Extremely enlarged orifice of the vestibular aqueduct (1) extending toward the sigmoid sinus (2). Furthermore, there is fusion of the second and third cochlear turns (3) and opacification of the mastoid and middle ear.

Internal Auditory Canal, Enlargements

Differential Diagnosis

- Congenital schwannoma of the auditory or facial nerve, extension of meningioma or arachnoid cysts into the internal auditory canal.
- Inflammatory processes with the formation of granulation tissue (e.g., otosyphilis; see also Chapter 5)
- Infiltrative processes such as endolymphatic sac tumor.

Points of Evaluation

- An internal auditory canal width of less than 3 mm is considered pathologic and may also indicate hypoplasia or absence of its contents.
- A width of more than 10 mm may also be pathologic, and assessment of the bony outline of the meatus is essential in the evaluation of pathology. Intralesional calcifications and hyperostosis are suggestive of meningioma.
- MRI is complementary to CT and is often decisive in making a correct (differential) diagnosis.
- Bilateral expanding lesions of the internal auditory canal are strongly suggestive of neurofibromatosis type II (see also Chapter 5).

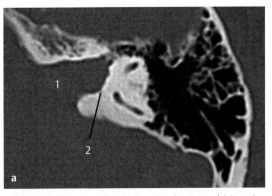

Fig. 3.34 a–c
Patient with progressive bilateral perceptive hearing loss.

a CT, axial. Widening of the internal auditory canal (1), with a slightly irregular bony outline (2) suggestive of an intrameatal process. In this patient, known to have neurofibromatosis type 2, a schwannoma was seen on MRI.

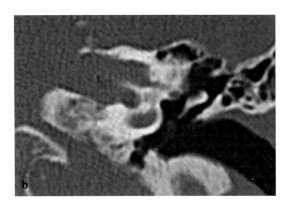

b CT, coronal. Same patient with a full-length, broadened appearance of the internal auditory canal (1) up to the region of the fundus of the cochlea.

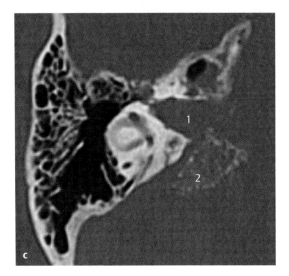

c CT, axial. The contralateral side of the same patient also shows widening of the internal auditory canal (1), with a slightly irregular bony outline. Furthermore, there are signs of calcifications (2) suggestive of meningioma.

Ossification of the Labyrinth after Meningitis

Differential Diagnosis
- Pneumococcal meningitis has the highest risk of inducing ossifications in the labyrinth.
- Any labyrinthitis that may result in ossification (see also next section, p. 82).

Points of Evaluation
In meningitis, the bacterial endotoxins released when antibiotics are administered cause damage to the inner ear neural structures. An inflammatory response is also induced in the labyrinth with resulting fibrosis and ossification within weeks to several months after treatment. In cases of bilateral and severe sensorineural hearing loss, these changes may interfere with cochlear implantation. CT and MRI with gadolinium enhancement are complementary and might reveal early changes of possible obliteration and/or ossification.

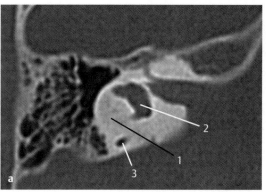

Fig. 3.35 a–c Patients with a history of meningitis.

a CT, axial. Due to a concomitant labyrinthitis, several months later the horizontal semicircular canal is completely ossified (1). The vestibule (2), and the posterior semicircular canal (3) are unaffected. The cochlea was unaffected (not shown), which made insertion of a cochlear implant (in case of bilateral and postlingual deafness) feasible.

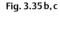

Fig. 3.35 b, c

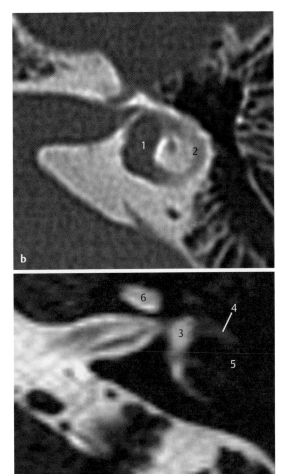

b, c CT and MRI T2-weighted, axial. In this patient, 2 years after meningitis, evaluation of the inner ear revealed normal appearance of the vestibule on CT (1). However, slight opacities in the horizontal semicircular canal were demonstrated (2), which might suggest fibrosis or ossification of its lumen. MRI confirmed normal inner ear fluid content of the vestibule (3). The horizontal canal shows moderate intensity in the anterior part of the canal (4), but the remaining parts of the canal are completely obliterated (5). Note also the normal fluid content of the basal cochlear turn (6), as well as the rest of the cochlea, which was also expected from the CT findings (not shown).

Labyrinthitis Ossificans

Differential Diagnosis

Any cause of labyrinthitis: pathogens (viral, bacterial), autoimmune, Cogan (with interstitial keratitis of the cornea), *Treponema pallidum* (otosyphilis). Post-traumatic labyrinthitis. Intralabyrinthine hemorrhage (due to trauma or concomitant by infection).

Points of Evaluation

- Labyrinthitis may arise by spread from a middle ear infection or its bacterial endotoxins (mostly unilateral), meningitis by the connections between the labyrinth and the cerebrospinal fluid (frequently bilateral), or by hematogenic spread. CT, MRI, and laboratory tests must be used to distinguish between these causes.
- Localized contrast enhancement on MRI might indicate an intralabyrinthine schwannoma (see also Chapter 5).
- Other clinical symptoms besides the inner ear symptoms are important to establish the most likely diagnosis (see also Chapter 5).

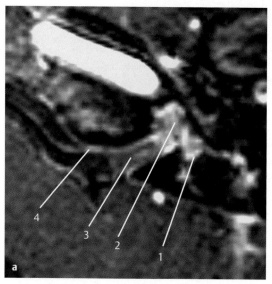

Fig. 3.36 a–c Patient presenting with unilateral sudden deafness due to otosyphilis.

a MRI, T1-weighted with gadolinium enhancement, axial. There is enhancement of the vestibule (1), cochlear contents (2), and the contents (3), as well as the dural outline (4) of the internal auditory canal. The patient was successfully treated with antibiotics.

Fig. 3.36 b, c

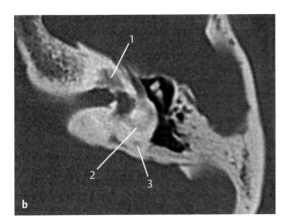

b CT, axial. Eight months later there is ossification of the basal cochlear turn (1) and the horizontal (2) and posterior (3) semicircular canals.

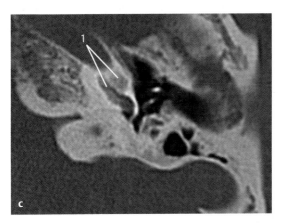

c CT, axial. An axial slice through the cochlea shows ossifications and probably fibrosis of the entire cochlea (1), from which the outlines are still visible.

Otosclerosis, Retrofenestral

Differential Diagnosis

- Other than otosclerosis, a condition that shows such bony changes of the otic capsule is mainly osteogenesis imperfecta with a clinical history of frequent fractures due to minor trauma everywhere in the body. These patients may have the typically blue sclerae.
- Furthermore, osseous dystrophies such as fibrous dysplasia or Paget disease must be kept in mind. As indicated in **Fig. 3.37c**, ossifications due to previous labyrinthitis may be considered.

Points of Evaluation

- Extension of demineralization. It may be unilateral or bilateral and may vary between both ears. Most cases of otosclerosis demonstrate minor deformities as described in "Pathology of the Middle Ear" earlier in this chapter.
- In cases of severe bilateral hearing disorders or complete deafness, cochlear implantation may be considered, although the patency of the cochlear lumen is essential for correct and complete electrode insertion. There is a risk of going down a false route due to the severe demineralization and distortion of the normal anatomy.

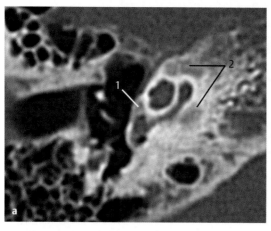

Fig. 3.37 a–c   Patient with conductive hearing loss and normal otoscopic findings.

a CT, axial. Fenestral otosclerosis as indicated by the lucent lesion at the fissula ante fenestram (1). Note the obvious **retrofenestral otosclerosis** as demonstrated by lucencies of the otic capsule around the cochlea (2), a so-called halo phenomenon or fourth ring of Valvassori.

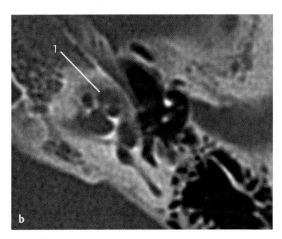

Fig. 3.37 b, c

b CT, axial. Another patient with more diffuse demineralization of the otic capsule (1). The delineation of the cochlear lumen is ill-defined.

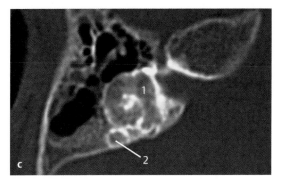

c CT, axial. Spongy appearance of the delineation and contents of the vestibule (1) and horizontal semicircular canal. The posterior canal is also affected (2). Ossification of the semicircular canals due to a previous labyrinthitis might also be considered in this case.

Osteogenesis Imperfecta

Differential Diagnosis
The condition that shows such bony changes of the otic capsule is mainly otosclerosis. Furthermore, osseous dystrophies such as fibrous dysplasia or Paget disease must be kept in mind.

Points of Evaluation
- Extension of demineralization, which may be unilateral or bilateral and may vary between both ears. Most cases of osteogenesis imperfecta have minor abnormalities as described in "Pathology of the Middle Ear" earlier in this chapter. A clinical history of frequent and multiple fractures due to minor trauma everywhere in the body, as well as the typical blue sclerae, might help make the diagnosis.
- In cases of severe bilateral hearing disorders or complete deafness, cochlear implantation may be considered, although the patency of the cochlear lumen is essential for correct and complete electrode insertion. There is the risk of going down a false route due to the severe demineralization and distortion of the normal anatomy.

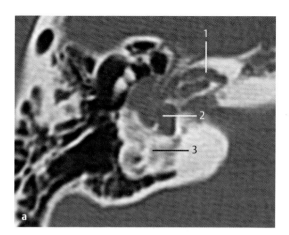

Fig. 3.38 a, b   Patient with osteogenesis imperfecta and progressive mixed hearing loss.

a CT, axial. Severe demineralization of the otic capsule around the cochlea (1), vestibule (2), and to a lesser degree, around the semicircular canals (3).

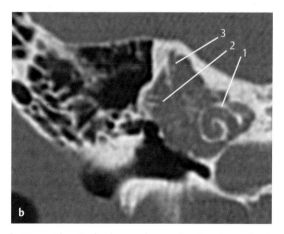

b CT, semi-longitudinal coronal reconstruction. Reconstructed view in the same patient as in **Fig. 3.38 a**. Only a small bony shell remains around the cochlea (1) and the horizontal (2) and the anterior (3) semicircular canals. The vestibule is grossly expanded and cannot be recognized.

Fibrous Dysplasia (2)

Differential Diagnosis
Localized at the dural outlines, these finding may also be suggestive of:
- Meningioma (see also Chapter 5).
- Paget disease (initial involvement of marrow-containing periosteal bone).
- Osteopetrosis (diffuse bony sclerosis without the increased volume of bone see in fibrous dysplasia).
- Extreme forms of otosclerosis (bound to the otic capsule).
- Osteogenesis imperfecta.

Points of Evaluation
- Radiologically on CT, enlargement of bone with intact cortical outlines and a dense "ground glass" appearance is characteristic of fibrous dysplasia. Fibrous dysplasia incidentally found on MRI may be confused with a malignancy.
- Fibrous dysplasia in a single osseous structure (monostotic) can be monitored with serial scanning and can be stable and asymptomatic for years.
- In cases of meningioma, the bony outlines can be irregular and hyperostosis can be found as well as a dural tail. Intracranial calcifications may be suggestive of a meningioma.

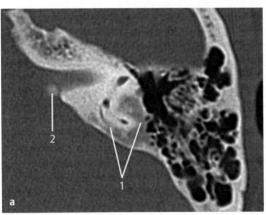

Fig. 3.39 a–c Patient evaluated for perceptive hearing loss of unknown origin.

a CT, axial. In the area of the posterior part of the labyrinth, around the posterior semicircular canal there is demineralization with a "ground glass" appearance (1), suggestive of an isolated area of fibrous dysplasia. Furthermore, an exophytic bony process is visible (2) at the margin of the internal auditory canal. Hyperostosis and calcifications, in combination with a lesion as seen around the semicircular canal, might indicate a meningioma, although the dural outlines seem to be unaffected.

Fig. 3.39 b, c

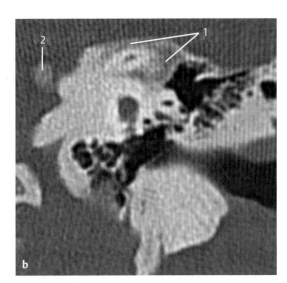

b CT, coronal. The demineralization around the semicircular canal (1) seems isolated from the exophytic bony process (2). No fistula was noted in the labyrinth. Biopsy confirmed the diagnosis of fibrous dysplasia.

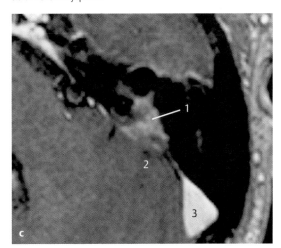

c MRI, T1-weighted with gadolinium enhancement, axial. The isolated localization of the lesion was confirmed at MRI (1), with mild contrast enhancement. No dural or intracranial involvement is demonstrated (2). Flow in the sigmoid sinus is present (3).

Cochlear Implantation

Some pathologies such as malformations, ossifications due to labyrinthitis or meningitis, and demineralization diseases such as otosclerosis and osteogenesis imperfecta may result in insertion problems as well as going down a false route. Below are some illustrative cases in which radiologic evaluation was helpful.

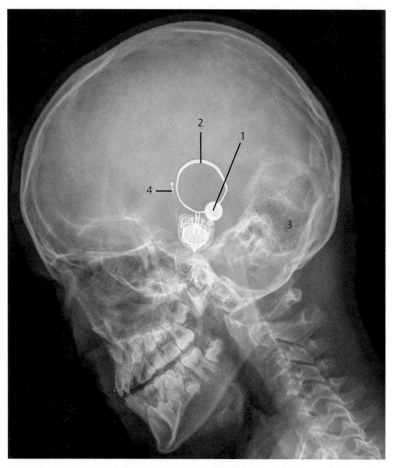

Fig. 3.40 Dysfunction of the cochlear implant after head trauma. Plain film, lateral skull view. This view demonstrates dislocation of the magnet (1) from its silicone sheet in the middle of the ring (2). The magnet is important for the fixation of the outer transmission coil and adequate transmission of energy and sound information. There is a clear view of the pneumatized and aerated mastoid (3) and the reference electrode (4). The intracochlear electrode is well positioned, although it is not very well seen on this view.

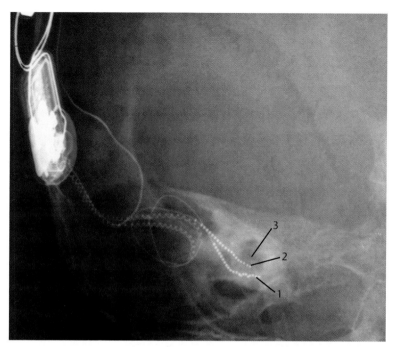

Fig. 3.41 **Patient with a history of meningitis and a split array because of technical problems at the time of insertion. Plain film, stenvers view.** The basal electrode (1) is partially introduced as well as the electrode in the middle turn (2). The insertion problems are the result of mild but obstructive ossification, as expected with preoperative CT. The apical turn (3) contains no electrode. Optimal hearing revalidation was not achieved in this patient.

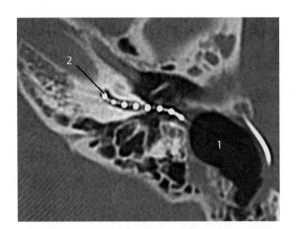

Fig. 3.42 Patient with a history of a bilateral petrositis and mastoiditis, resulting in bilateral deafness.

CT, axial. A mastoidectomy was performed to drain the infection (1). At a later stage, a cochlear implant was inserted in the basal turn of the cochlea (2). The middle and superior cochlear turns show ossification, which was found preoperatively and on this postoperative CT. Hearing results were quite poor, probably due to this partial implantation as well as possible auditory nerve pathology.

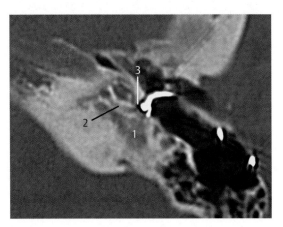

Fig. 3.43 Patient with osteogenesis imperfecta and severe demineralization of the otic capsule resulting in bilateral deafness.

CT, axial. At surgery, the perilymphatic space was difficult to find as a result of changes due to demineralization around the cochlea (1) and intraluminal ossifications in the basal turn (2). As a result, the electrode could not be inserted deeply but was placed just at the basal turn (3), without satisfactory results.

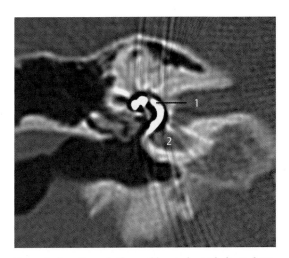

Fig. 3.44 Patient with electrode dysfunction after cochlear implantation.

Coronal view through the cochlea and vestibule. Unfortunately, the electrode has been inserted in the vestibule (1) instead of the cochlea (2), probably due to fibrosis or a wrong angle of insertion through the cochleostomy. No ossifications of the basal turn were observed. Hearing results were poor and a reimplantation was carried out.

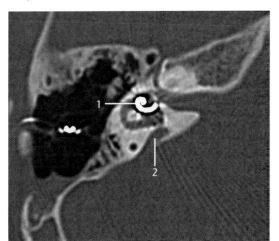

Fig. 3.45 Patient with electrode dysfunction after cochlear implantation.

CT, axial. Another example of insertion in the vestibule (1). In this patient, a common cavity of the cochlea was present, with an increased risk of misplacement. The enlarged vestibular aqueduct (2) is a frequently found comorbidity in labyrinthine anomalies.

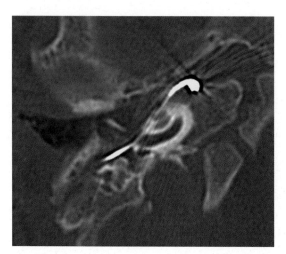

Fig. 3.46 Patient with perioperative difficulties of implantation.

CT, axial. The intracochlear lumen was difficult to find due to mucosal thickening. After finding a lumen suggestive of the perilymphatic space, insertion was easy. Perioperative measurements did not show adequate responses. Postoperative CT shows misplacement of the electrode in the carotid canal. A perioperative Stenvers could have confirmed misplacement. At a later stage, reimplantation was performed without complications and with good hearing results.

Skull Base

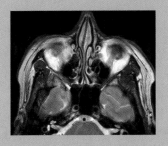

4 Radiologic Anatomy of the Skull Base

The skull base can be evaluated by computed tomography (CT), which will demonstrate the bony structures of the skull base with its foramina and fissures for vessels and cranial nerves, the temporal bone, and sinonasal cavities. Magnetic resonance imaging (MRI) will demonstrate the contents of the foramina and fissures as well as the intracranial soft tissues. CT or MRI may provide enough information individually to demonstrate and classify the pathology in this area, however, when used together these modalities can be complementary and define even better the invasion and destruction of (bony) structures of the skull base by soft-tissue masses.

Radiologic Evaluation Points of the Skull Base

Computed Tomography

- Bony outline of the outer skull.
- Bony outline of the intracranial skull base.
- Temporal bone structures: internal auditory canal, vestibular and cochlear aqueduct, apex.
- Foramina: ovale, spinosum, jugular, rotundum.
- Large vessels: carotid artery, sigmoid sinus, jugular bulb.
- Supraorbital fissure and orbital structures.
- Infratemporal fossa, sphenoidal bone, clivus.
- Clinoid processes, sella and pituitary fossa.
- Features of the pathology: expanding or invasive growth pattern.

Magnetic Resonance Imaging

- Intracranial brain structures: cerebrum, cerebellum, pons and brainstem, ventricles, dural outlines.
- Vascular structures: transverse sinus, sigmoid sinus and jugular bulb, superior petrosal sinus, carotid artery, vertebrobasilar system, anterior and posterior inferior cerebellar arteries (AICA and PICA).
- Temporal bone: fluid contents (T2-weighted MR image) of inner ear structures and internal auditory canal, appearance of the cochlear, vestibular (inferior and superior), and facial nerves.

- Other cranial nerves: olfactory region, optic nerve, supraorbital fissure, abducens and trigeminal nerves, Meckel cave.
- Intensities on T1-weighted and T2-weighted MR images, with contrast, and possible asymmetry.

Evaluation of the Skull Base on Axial CT Slices in a Craniocaudal Sequence

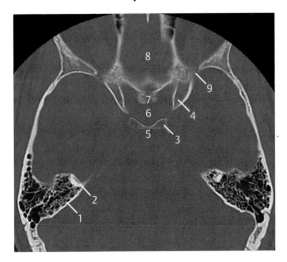

Fig. 4.1   CT slice.
1 Temporal bone
2 Anterior semicircular canal
3 Posterior clinoid
4 Anterior clinoid
5 Dorsum sellae
6 Pituitary fossa
7 Tuberculum sellae
8 Fovea ethmoidalis (cranial nerve I in anterior cranial fossa)
9 Superior orbital fissure

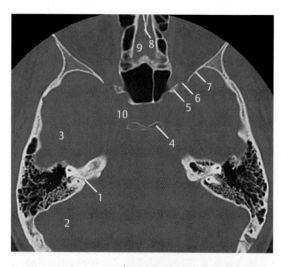

Fig. 4.2   Axial CT slice.
1 Subarcuate canal and artery
2 Posterior cranial fossa
3 Middle cranial fossa
4 Posterior clinoid process
5 Anterior clinoid process
6 Superior orbital fissure (cranial nerves III, IV, VI, and a part of V)
7 Sphenoid bone
8 Crista galli
9 Fovea ethmoidalis
10 Region of the cavernous sinus and internal carotid artery

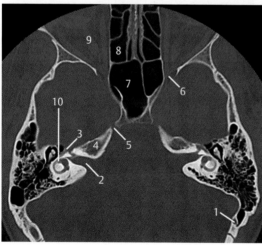

Fig. 4.3   Axial CT slice.
1 Emissary vein
2 Internal auditory canal (cranial nerves VII and VIII)
3 Geniculate ganglion
4 Petrous apex
5 Foramen for the ophthalmic nerve (part of the trigeminal nerve)
6 Superior orbital fissure
7 Sphenoid sinus
8 Ethmoid sinus
9 Optic nerve (cranial nerve II)
10 Horizontal semicircular canal and vestibule

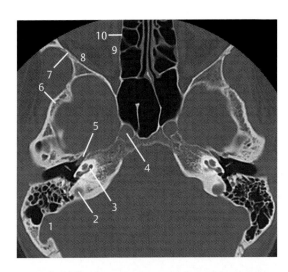

Fig. 4.4 Axial CT slice.
1 Sigmoid sinus
2 Roof of the jugular bulb
3 Cochlea (basal turn)
4 Internal carotid artery
5 Eustachian tube
6 Temporal bone (squamous part)
7 Greater wing of sphenoid
8 Lateral rectus
9 Medial rectus
10 Lamina papyracea

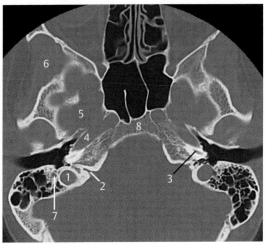

Fig. 4.5 Axial CT slice.
1 Jugular bulb
2 Cochlear aqueduct
3 Basal turn of cochlea
4 Internal carotid artery
5 Middle cranial fossa
6 Infratemporal fossa
7 Facial nerve (cranial nerve VII)
8 Clivus

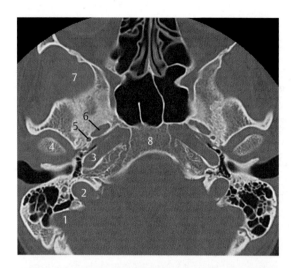

Fig. 4.6 Axial CT slice.
1 Sigmoid sinus
2 Jugular bulb
3 Internal carotid artery
4 Mandibular condyle
5 Foramen spinosum
6 Foramen ovale (mandibular part of the trigeminal nerve)
7 Infratemporal fossa
8 Clivus

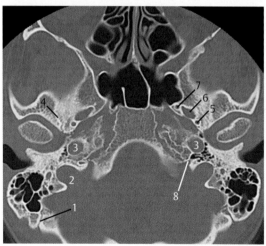

Fig. 4.7 Axial CT slice.
1 Occipitomastoid suture
2 Jugular bulb
3 Internal carotid artery
4 Sphenosquamosal suture
5 Foramen spinosum
6 Foramen ovale (mandibular part of the trigeminal nerve)
7 Foramen rotundum (maxillary part of the trigeminal nerve)
8 Jugular foramen (cranial nerves IX, X, and XI)

Evaluation of the Skull Base on Coronal CT Slices in an Anteroposterior Sequence

(See also Chapter 2 for anatomy of the temporal bone.)

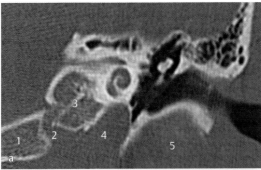
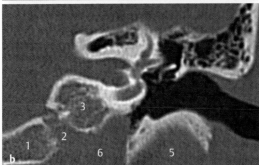
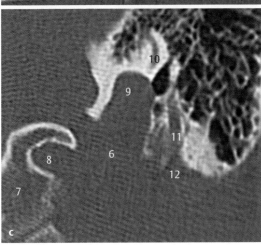

Fig. 4.8 a–c   Coronal CT slices.

1 Clivus
2 Occipitomastoidal suture
3 Base of petrous bone
4 Internal carotid artery
5 Region of the temporomandibular joint
6 Jugular foramen
7 Occipital condyle
8 Hypoglossal canal (cranial nerve XII)
9 Jugular bulb
10 Posterior semi-circular canal
11 Mastoid portion of the facial nerve (cranial nerve VII)
12 Stylomastoid foramen (cranial nerve VII)

Evaluation of the Middle and Posterior Cranial Fossae on Axial MRI Slices in a Craniocaudal Sequence

(Labeled structures may be present on other slices without being labeled again.)

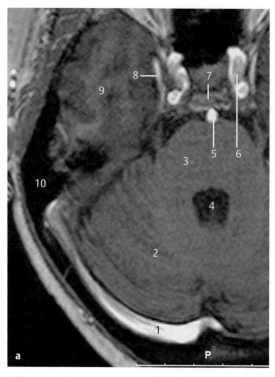

Fig. 4.9 a–c   Axial slices of the same level: T1-weighted MR image without contrast (a), T1-weighted MR image with gadolinium enhancement (b), and T2-weighted MR image (c).

1 Transverse sinus
2 Cerebellum
3 Pons
4 Fourth ventricle
5 Basilar artery
6 Internal carotid artery
7 Dorsum sellae
8 Anterior cerebral artery
9 Temporal lobe
10 Pneumatized and aerated mastoidal cells
11 Mastoidal emissary vein
12 Sigmoid sinus
13 Superior petrosal sinus
14 Cavernous sinus
15 Optic nerve (cranial nerve II)
16 Superior semicircular canal

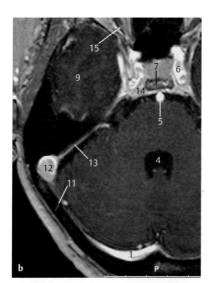

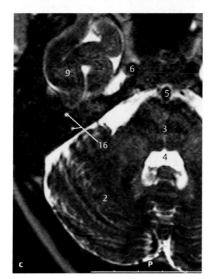

Fig. 4.9 b, c

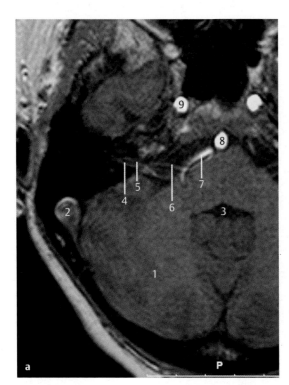

Fig. 4.10 a–c Axial slices of the same level: T1-weighted MR image without contrast (a), T1-weighted MR image with gadolinium enhancement (b), and T2-weighted MR image (c).

1 Cerebellum
2 Sigmoid sinus
3 Fourth ventricle
4 Vestibular nerve (cranial nerve VIII)
5 Cochlear nerve (cranial nerve VIII)
6 Anterior inferior cerebellar artery (AICA)
7 Probably posterior inferior cerebellar artery (PICA), although a lower course is more common
8 Basilar artery

9 Internal carotid artery
10 Fluid content of the posterior semicircular canal
11 Fluid content of the horizontal semicircular canal and vestibule
12 Fluid content of the basal turn of the cochlea
13 Cerebrospinal fluid
14 Facial nerve (cranial nerve VII)
15 Abducens nerve (cranial nerve VI)

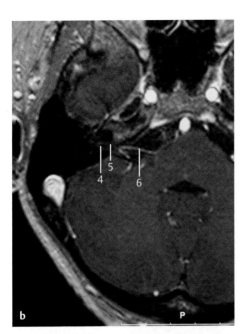

Fig. 4.10 b, c

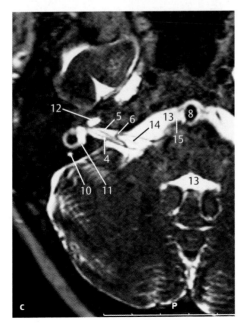

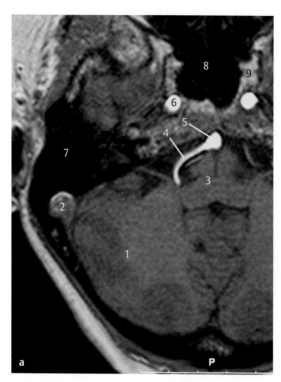

Fig. 4.11 a–c Axial slices of the same level: T1-weighted MR image without contrast (a), T1-weighted MR image with gadolinium enhancement (b), and T2-weighted MR image (c).

1 Cerebellum
2 Sigmoid sinus
3 Ponto-medullary transition
4 Probably posterior inferior cerebellar artery (PICA, originating from the vertebral artery)
5 Basilar artery
6 Internal carotid artery
7 Pneumatized and aerated mastoidal cells
8 Sphenoid sinus
9 Cavernous sinus
10 Probably anterior inferior cerebellar artery (AICA)
11 Fluid content of the posterior semicircular canal
12 Fluid content of the vestibule
13 Cochlear fluid contents

Fig. 4.11 b, c

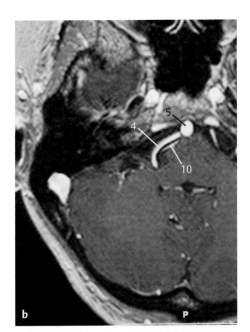

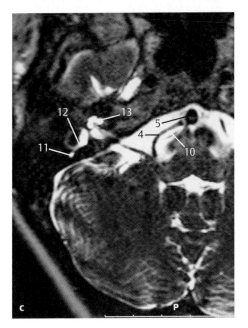

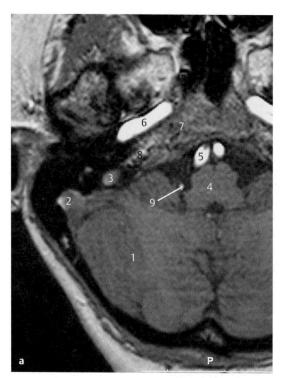

Fig. 4.12 a–c Axial slices of the same level: T1-weighted MR image without contrast (a), T1-weighted MR image with gadolinium enhancement (b), and T2-weighted MR image (c).

1 Cerebellum
2 Sigmoid sinus
3 Roof of the jugular bulb
4 Medulla
5 Vertebral artery
6 Internal carotid artery
7 Clivus (bone marrow content)
8 Petrosal apex (bone marrow content)
9 Posterior inferior cerebellar artery (PICA)

Fig. 4.12 b, c

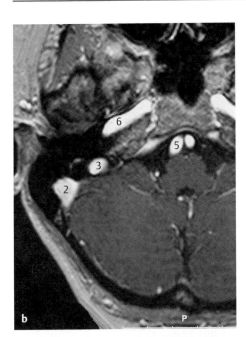

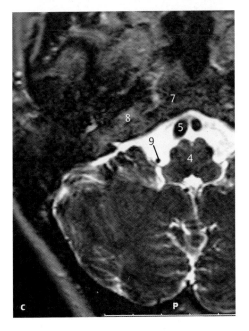

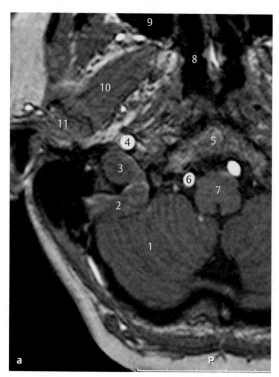

Fig. 4.13 a–c   Axial slices of the same level: T1-weighted MR image without contrast (a), T1-weighted MR image with gadolinium enhancement (b), and T2-weighted MR image (c).

1 Cerebellum
2 Jugular bulb
3 Jugular vein
4 Internal carotid artery
5 Clivus
6 Vertebral artery

7 Medulla
8 Nasal lumen (air space)
9 Maxillary sinus
10 Lateral pterygoid
11 Mandibular condyle
12 Cerebrospinal fluid

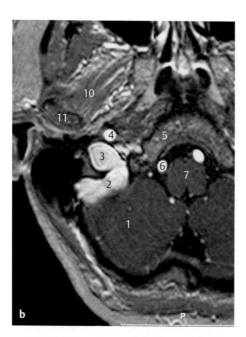

Fig. 4.13 b, c

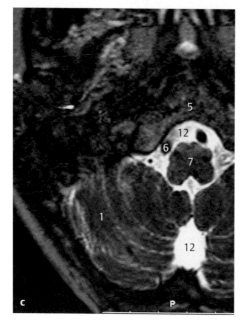

Miscellaneous Skull Base Views

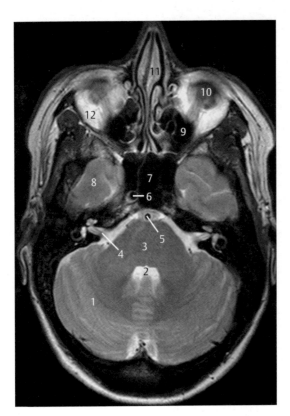

Fig. 4.14 Axial overview of the skull base on MRI.
1 Cerebellum
2 Fourth ventricle
3 Brainstem
4 Internal auditory canal
5 Basilar artery
6 Internal carotid artery
7 Sphenoid sinus
8 Temporal lobe
9 Ethmoid sinus
10 Eyeball
11 Nasal septum
12 Orbital fat

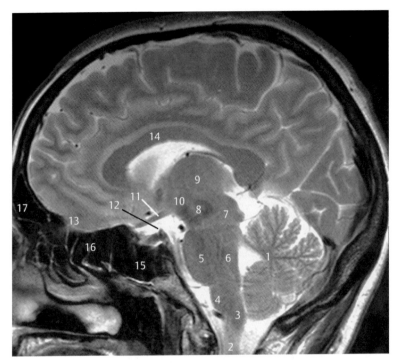

Fig. 4.15 Sagittal overview of the skull on MRI.

1 Cerebellum (arbor vitae)
2 Medulla
3 Nucleus cuneatus
4 Nucleus olivaris
5 Nucleus pontis and tract
6 Tegmentum pontis
7 Lemniscus medialis and tegmentum mesencephali
8 Mesencephalon
9 Thalamus
10 Hypothalamus
11 Optic chiasma (cranial nerve II)
12 Pituitary fossa
13 Olfactory bulb (cranial nerve I)
14 Corpus callosum
15 Sphenoid sinus
16 Ethmoid sinus
17 Frontal sinus

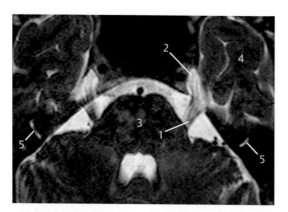

Fig. 4.16 Trigeminal nerve.

MRI, T2-weighted, axial. View on the trigeminal nerve (1), and the trigeminal ganglion in the Meckel cave (2). The nerve derives from the pons (3). Also seen are the temporal lobe (4) and superior part of the anterior semicircular canal (5). Distal to the ganglion, the nerve divides into three parts: the ophthalmic nerve, which exits through the superior orbital fissure; the maxillary nerve, which exits through the foramen rotundum; and the mandibular nerve, which exits through the foramen ovale.

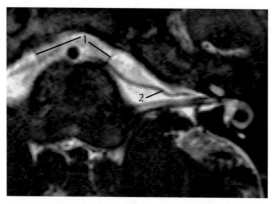

Fig. 4.17 Abducens nerve.

MRI, T2-weighted, axial. The abducens, deriving from the pons, is bilaterally visible in its anterior passage (1) through the cerebrospinal fluid. Also seen is the anterior inferior cerebellar artery (2) coursing through the cerebrospinal fluid to the cerebellopontine angle with a loop into the internal auditory canal.

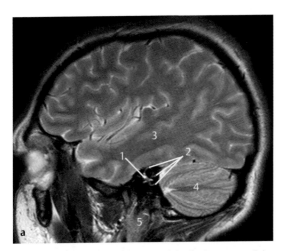

Fig. 4.18 a, b   Sagittal view of the inner ear structures.

a MRI, T2-weighted, sagittal. View of the fluid contents of the vestibule (1) and semicircular canals (2) between the cerebrum (3), cerebellum (4), and pons (5).

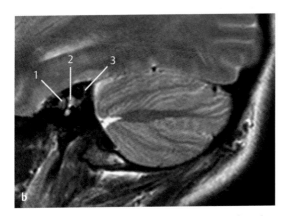

b MRI, T2-weighted, axial. Close-up view of another slice shows the fluid contents of the cochlear turns (1), vestibule (2), and the posterior semicircular canal (3).

5 Pathology of the Skull Base

Pathology of the Middle Skull Base

Lesions in the cerebellopontine angle (CPA) may be evaluated as shown in **Table 5.1**, according to intensity (T1/T2-weighted), contrast enhancement, and commonly occurring or characteristic radiologic features. Then, in combination with the clinical symptoms, the most likely diagnosis can be made. Note that **Table 5.1** is not comprehensive and variations in presentation maybe seen. A variety of CPA pathologies will be discussed in this chapter.

Table 5.1 Differential diagnosis of lesions in the cerebellopontine angle (CPA)

Intensity T1W	T2Wa	Contrast enhancement	Radiologic characteristics	Clinical characteristics	Diagnosis
Hypo/iso	Hypo	Yes	Dural hypertrophy, often thin and hyperintense lining	Meningeal symptoms, headaches, fever, drowsiness, cranial nerve dysfunction	Pachymeningitis
Hypo	Hypo	Variable	Flow voids on T1 and T2	Female:male ratio: 2:1	Aneurysm
Hypo	Hypo	Variable	Flow voids on T1 and T2, elongation, sometimes dolicho basilar artery	Cranial nerve or brainstem compression: trigeminal neuralgia, hemifacial spasm. Obstruction hydrocephalus	Arteriovenous malformation
Hypo	Hyper	Variable	Exophytic aspect, brain stem expansion	Rapidly progressive clinical symptomatology, motor dysfunction, headaches and visual impairment	Astrocytoma
Hypo	Hyper	Variable	Heterogeneous signal, calcifications, hypointense lining of hemosiderin	Early facial dysfunction, sometimes hormone-related, progression during pregnancy	Cavernous hemangioma

Table 5.1 Differential diagnosis of lesions in the cerebellopontine angle (CPA) (cont.)

Intensity T1W	T2W[a]	Contrast enhancement	Radiologic characteristics	Clinical characteristics	Diagnosis
Hypo	Hyper	No	Irregular, lobulated, inclusion of blood vessels	5% of all CPA lesions, progressive cranial nerve V, VII, and cerebellar dysfunction	Epidermoid cyst
Hypo	Hyper	No	Cystic, vascular compressions	Same symptomatology but less frequent than in epidermoid cysts, often asymptomatic	Arachnoidal cyst
Hypo	Hyper	Yes	Near petro-occipital fissure, hyperintense lining, calcifications, hypointense on CT	Cochleovestibular dysfunction, headaches, hematoma in pons, cranial nerve III dysfunction	Chondroma
Hypo	Hyper	Yes	Near petro-occipital fissure, hyperintense lining, calcifications, hypointense on CT	See also chondroma, sometimes also diplopia and cranial nerve V dysfunction	Chondrosarcoma
Hypo	Hyper	Yes	Lobulated, irregular bony erosions, calcifications around tumor lining	Often cranial nerve VI dysfunction, facial neuralgia and ataxia, male:female ratio: 2:1	Chordoma
Hypo	Hyper	Yes	Enhancing solid mass around sella turcica, sometimes expanding into the sphenoid sinus	Visual impairment, Cushing, diabetes insipidus, hyperthyroid dysfunction	Pituitary gland adenoma
Hypo	Hyper	Yes	Ice cone lesion in the CPA, distended cisternal space, intra- and extracanalicular growth	Slow growth pattern and late symptomatology, 70–80% of all CPA lesions	Schwannoma

Continued on next page

Table 5.1 Differential diagnosis of lesions in the cerebellopontine angle (CPA) (cont.)

Intensity T1W	T2W[a]	Contrast enhancement	Radiologic characteristics	Clinical characteristics	Diagnosis
Hypo	Hyper	Yes	Strongly enhancing homogeneous mass	Related to immune suppression, relatively fast growing	Lymphoma
Hypo	Hyper	Yes	Lobulated, calcifications, focal bleedings, vessel ingrowth, often hydrocephalus	Originates from choroid plexus in the fourth ventricle. Headaches, papillary edema, vomiting	Papilloma
Hypo	Hyper	Yes	Depending on primary tumor, peritumoral edema	Often multiple lesions, oncologic history	Metastasis
Hypo	Hyper	Yes	Homogeneous cystic mass with a high vascularity	Associated with Von Hippel–Lindau disease, sometimes cerebellar ataxia	Hemangioblastoma
Hypo	Hyper	Yes	Rounded or oval homogeneous appearance, irregular lining between tumor and brain	Neuroepithelial tumor frequently in children, often metastasis along neuraxis	Medulloblastoma
Hypo	Hyper	Yes	Irregular lobulated, isointense, microcysts, necrosis and hemorrhages, calcifications on CT	Often growth from fourth ventricle, sometimes headaches and papillary edema	Ependymoma
Hypo	Hyper	Yes	Salt and pepper configuration due to intratumoral hemorrhage/flow voids, spiculated aspect on CT	Often originates from the glomus tympanicum or jugulare, sometimes conductive hearing loss	Paraganglioma
Hypo	Hyper	Yes	Enhancing destructive opacities in petrous apex, middle ear effusion	Severe otalgia, in case of Gradenigo syndrome: cranial nerve V or cranial nerve VI dysfunction, conductive hearing losses	Apical petrositis

Table 5.1 Differential diagnosis of lesions in the cerebellopontine angle (CPA) (cont.)

Intensity T1W	T2W[a]	Contrast enhancement	Radiologic characteristics	Clinical characteristics	Diagnosis
Hyper	Fat iso	No	Hyperintense, homogeneous signal, decreased intensity after fat suppression	Cochleovestibular dysfunction by pressure	Lipoma
Hyper	Hypo/iso	Yes	Homogeneous lesion, similar to meningioma, often in meningeal region	Often metastasis, sometimes increased intracranial pressure and meningism	Melanoma
Hyper	Hypo	No	Heterogeneous, often cystic appearance	Very rare, 50% of the teratomas are found in neonates	Teratoma
Hyper	Hypo	No	Avascular irregular, lobulated mass, peripheral calcifications on CT	Few cochleovestibular complaints, headaches and cranial nerve V and IX dysfunction	Dermoid cyst
Hyper	Hypo	Yes	Enhancement inside the labyrinth, beware of opacities in the temporal bone	Severe and acute vertigo, hearing loss and tinnitus, possible viral or bacterial pathogens	Labyrinthitis
Hyper	Hyper	No	Expansive lytic lesion anterior to the petrous apex, hypointense lining	Often starting with cochleovestibular complaints, sometimes middle ear involvement	Cholesterol-granuloma
Variable	Hyper	Yes	Cystic, highly vascularized and protein-rich, some flow voids, infiltrative spread to temporal bone/intracranial	Frequently starting with cochleovestibular complaints or facial nerve dysfunction, blue mass behind the ear drum	Endolymphatic sac tumor

Continued on next page

Table 5.1   Differential diagnosis of lesions in the cerebellopontine angle (CPA) (cont.)

Intensity T1W	T2W[a]	Contrast enhance-ment	Radiologic characteristics	Clinical characteristics	Diagnosis
Iso	Hypo	No	Lobulated mass, often in subarach-noidal spaces with marginal hypo-intensities	Progressive percep-tive hearing loss, cerebellar ataxia, pyramidal symp-toms	Siderosis
Iso	Hypo	Yes	Diffuse plaques in and around the meninges	Neurologic deficits, cranial nerve dys-function, in combi-nation with pulmo-nary lesions	(Neuro) sarcoidosis
Iso	Hyper	Yes	Hemispheric tu-mor with dural tail, sometimes calcifications and flow voids	Nystagmus, ataxia, 10–15% of all CPA lesions	Meningioma
Variable	Variable	Variable	Calcifications in cases of resorp-tion	History of trauma to the head	Hematoma

[a] Conventional T2 view; in constructive interference steady state (CISS) images (fluid maximal hyper-intense), the process is visualized as a hypointense lesion.

Pseudotumors in the Apex of the Petrous Bone

Differential Diagnosis
Hemangioma, cholesterol cyst (granuloma), cholesteatoma, epidermoid, and lymphangioma.

Points of Evaluation
- Pseudotumors of the petrous apex are often found incidentally owing to normal variations in anatomy. It is important to be aware of their harmless nature and to reassure the patient.
- Hemangiomas demonstrate a salt and pepper configuration, although they are rare in the petrous apex.
- A cholesterol cyst (granuloma) is hyperintense on T2-weighted images due to mucus stasis, and hyperintense on T1-weighted images due to hemorrhagic changes with possible contrast enhancement of the capsule and expansive characteristics.
- Cholesteatoma appears less bright on T1-weighted images.
- Epidermoids demonstrate hypointense T1- and hyperintense T2-weighted signal intensity.
- For lymphangioma, see separate section.

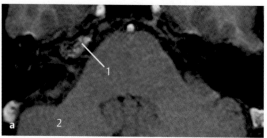

Fig. 5.1 a–c Patient with tinnitus, who was referred from another hospital with a mass in the region of the right petrous apex.

a MRI, T1-weighted, axial. T1-weighted image shows that the lesion (1) has high signal intensity compared with brain tissue (2). The contralateral petrous apex has low signal intensity. With gadolinium administration (not shown) no enhancement was seen.

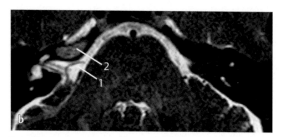

b MRI, T2-weighted, axial. On this heavily T2-weighted image, fluid (for example the cerebrospinal fluid [1] in the cerebellopontine cistern) has high signal intensity. The lesion (2) has slightly higher signal intensity than the brain tissue but not as high as fluid. Combined with the information from the T1-weighted image, this is a classic case of a pseudotumor due to asymmetric pneumatization of the petrous apex. The right petrous apex contains fatty marrow (high signal intensity on T1-weighted images), whereas the pneumatized contralateral apex only contains air with low signal intensity on both T1- and T2-weighted images.

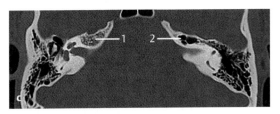

Fig. 5.1 c

c CT, axial. CT of the same patient confirms the difference in pneumatization and, in particular the aeration, of the petrous apex. **Note:** Normal bone marrow is present in the right petrous apex (1). Pneumatized petrous apex on the left side (2).

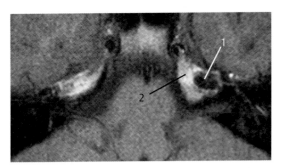

Fig. 5.2   Patient with perceptive hearing loss on the left side. Evaluation was done to exclude retrocochlear pathology.

MRI, T1-weighted, axial. A lesion (1) in the petrous apex on the left side. This type of lesions that appear black on T1-weighted sequences with or without contrast, as well as on T2-weighted sequences are indicative of **bone** or **aerated petrous cells**. On this image, the (remaining) petrous apex is filled with fatty marrow (2).

Schwannoma of the Internal Auditory Canal

Differential Diagnosis

Vestibular schwannoma, facial schwannoma, vascular tumors, inflammatory processes such as meningitis, neuritis, and gummas. Rare: meningioma, lipoma, metastases, lymphoma.

Points of Evaluation

- Vestibular schwannoma is the most frequent pathology (90%) found in this area. The clinical presentation facilitates the diagnosis because of hearing problems (vestibulocochlear).
- Multiple cranial nerve deficits are suggestive of inflammatory processes.
- A meningioma with the internal auditory canal as its only location and site of origin is possible but extremely rare; these tumors are usually CPA lesions protruding into the canal. In cases of a suspicious lesion in the CPA, MRI with contrast enhancement is recommended.

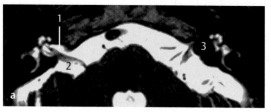

Fig. 5.3 a–c   Patient with slowly progressive left-sided sensorineural hearing loss.

a MRI, T2-weighted, axial. On this T2-weighted image, the cerebrospinal fluid has very high signal intensity. Normally, the internal auditory canal (1) and cerebellopontine angle/cistern (2) are filled with cerebrospinal fluid, whereas neural structures (i.e., vestibulocochlear and facial nerves) are seen as hypointense structures. The inner ear also displays high signal intensity due to the presence of fluid in the inner ear. However, in this patient a mass is present on the left side (3) in the internal auditory canal, which is partially obscuring the normal fluid contents, with some remaining fluid in the fundus of the inner ear. The contours are smooth, suggestive of a benign space-occupying lesion.

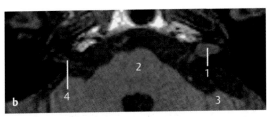

Fig. 5.3 b, c

b MRI, T1-weighted, axial. This T1-weighted image shows the lesion located in the left internal auditory canal, which is iso-intense to the brainstem (2) and cerebellum (3). Normal contents of the internal auditory canal (4) are less well visualized compared with the T2-weighted sequence. Compare with **Fig. 5.3 a**.

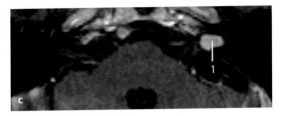

c MRI, T1-weighted with gadolinium enhancement, axial. Although the presence of a schwannoma in this region is highly likely, the use of gadolinium helps to confirm the diagnosis because schwannomas typically show strong homogeneous enhancement (1).

Vestibular Schwannoma

(For differential diagnosis and points of evaluation, see Cochlear Schwannoma

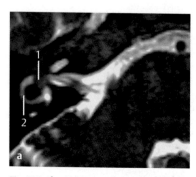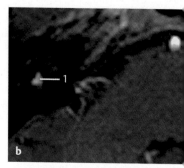

Fig. 5.4 a, b Patient with hearing deficits on the right side and nonspecific vertigo.

a MRI, T2-weighted, axial. A partial lack of fluid in the vestibule and horizontal semicircular canals is evident (1). A mass lesion is present in the vestibule. The status of the horizontal semicircular canal is unclear since it there is only reduced fluid content, as shown by its lowered signal intensity (2) and no definite mass.

b MRI, T1-weighted with gadolinium enhancement, axial. There is strong enhancement of the vestibule (1), which is highly suggestive of a vestibular schwannoma. The horizontal canal does not show any enhancement. A clear explanation of the hearing deficits could not be provided in this patient, since there was no involvement of the fundus.

Cochlear Schwannoma

Differential Diagnosis
Besides a high chance of schwannomas: inflammatory or immunological processes, secondary calcifications, congenital deformities of the inner ear.

Points of Evaluation
- Subtle and diffuse enhancements are also suggestive of active immunologic pathologies or intralabyrinthine infections.
- Fibrosis or ossification may occur over a period of months, excluding the possibility of cochlear implantation in bilateral deafness.
- CT may be able to differentiate between intraluminal fibrosis and ossification.

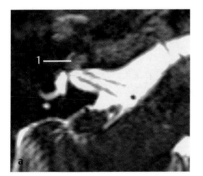 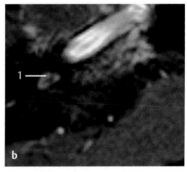

Fig. 5.5 a, b   Patient presenting with sudden deafness on the right side.

a MRI, T2-weighted, axial. MRI is a standard investigation in sudden deafness and revealed lack of fluid inside the cochlea (1). The vestibular parts of the inner ear and the internal auditory canal were normal.

b MRI, T1-weighted with gadolinium enhancement. The entire cochlea shows slight enhancement (1). Since there were no signs of infection clinically as well as on laboratory testing, the findings are highly suggestive of an intracochlear schwannoma.

Schwannoma of the Cerebellopontine Angle

Differential Diagnosis
Vestibular schwannoma, facial schwannoma, vascular tumors, inflammatory processes such as meningitis, neuritis, and gumma. Rare: lipoma, metastases, lymphoma.

Points of Evaluation
- A vestibular schwannoma is the most frequent pathology (90%) in this area. Its initial clinical presentation will help to determine the origin of the lesion, that is of hearing problems (vestibulocochlear) or facial paresis.
- Meningioma may show the so-called dural tail, although this is not always present, and involvement of the internal auditory canal is less common.
- Epidermoid cysts have a more rounded appearance, with contents which may also be hyperintense on T1-weighted images, but show lack of enhancement after contrast administration.
- Arachnoid cysts in the CPA may be confused with cystic tumors.
- Anterior localization may also indicate a trigeminal neurinoma.

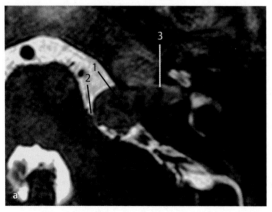

Fig. 5.6 a, b Patient with slowly progressive unilateral perceptive hearing loss.

a T2-weighted MRI, axial. Lesion of moderate size (1), partly within the internal auditory canal, and partly in the CPA, just touching the brainstem (2). Although the lateral part (fundus) of the internal auditory canal is not clearly filled with fluid, some still seems to be present (3) with the tumor restricted to the medial part of the canal.

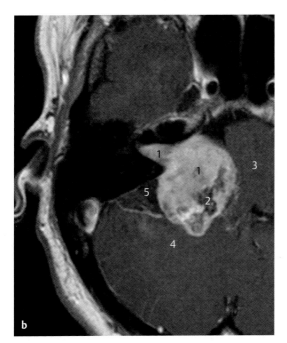

Fig. 5.6 b   Patient presenting with subacute unilateral deafness.

b MRI, T1-weighted with gadolinium enhancement, axial.
Example of a more extensive vestibulocochlear schwannoma.
The enhancing tumor is filling the internal auditory canal with a
large extension into the CPA (1). Due to the strong enhancement and location of the tumor, the findings are highly suggestive of a vestibulocochlear schwannoma. Nonenhancing areas
(2) most probably represent cystic degeneration, which is
often found in larger schwannomas. Note the compression of the
brainstem (3) and cerebellum (4). A subtle dural tail sign is present, which is more characteristic of meningioma. Posteriorly, an
arachnoid cyst may be present (5); this occasionally is the result
of an accumulation of cerebrospinal fluid due to occlusion and
mass effects by the tumor.

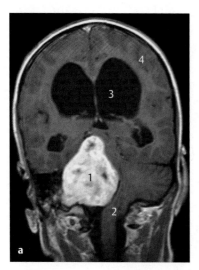

Fig. 5.7 a–d This 9-year old boy with intellectual disability was seen by several otolaryngologists over many years, who ascribed the hearing losses to retraction pockets of the ear drum, until raised intracranial pressure caused neurological deficits.

a T1-weighted MRI with gadolinium, coronal. Same schwannoma (1) with some cystic components, this image shows its superior extension and the severe compression and displacement of the brainstem (2). The dilated ventricles (3) indicate hydrocephalus due to obstruction with loss of the normal cortical appearance (4).

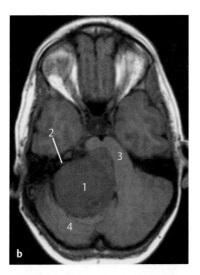

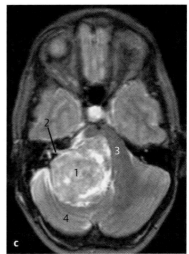

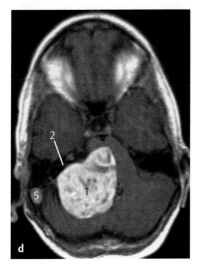

Fig. 5.7 b–d MRI, T1-weighted (b), T2-weighted (c), and T1-weighted with gadolinium enhancement (d), axial. Huge mass in the CPA (1) hypointense on T1-weighted imaging, mainly hyperintense on T2-weighted imaging, with gadolinium enhancement. No contrast enhancement is observed in the internal auditory canal. Although this is less typical of a schwannoma, it does not exclude this diagnosis because of its characteristics and rounded appearance. There is severe compression of the brainstem (3) and cerebellum (4) and enhancement of the contents of the right sigmoid sinus (5) which, in combination with the hyperintense T1-weighted image, is suggestive of sigmoid sinus thrombosis.

Arachnoid Cysts

Differential Diagnosis

Epidermoid cysts, cholesterol granuloma, cystic vestibular schwannoma. Rare: cysticercosis, congenital cysts.

Points of Evaluation

- Epidermoid cysts, which are also hypointense on T1-weighted sequences and hyperintense on T2-weighted sequences, can be differentiated with diffusion-weighted imaging (DWI).
- In contrast, lipomas are hyperintense on T1-weighted images and hypointense on spin-echo T2-weighted sequences.
- Cysticercosis is seen in endemic areas, and the lesions are often smaller in size.

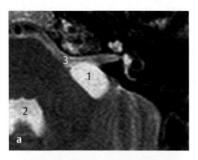

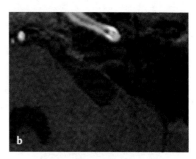

Fig. 5.8 a–e   Patients evaluated for complaints of disabling tinnitus.

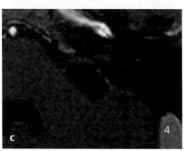

a–c MRI, T2-weighted (a), T1-weighted (b), and T1-weighted with gadolinium enhancement (c), axial. There is a smooth-bordered ovoid lesion (1) in the CPA, just posterior to the internal meatus of the internal auditory canal. The signal intensity of this lesion is comparable with the fluid in the fourth ventricle (2) and cerebellopontine cistern (3) on both the T2- and the T1-weighted images. On T1-weighted imaging with gadolinium enhancement, the sigmoid sinus enhances (4) but there is no enhancement of the lesion. On the basis of these image characteristics, the differential diagnosis is restricted to an arachnoid cyst. Arachnoid cysts may compress structures, resulting in neurologic deficits, but an exact relation with the clinical symptoms remains unclear in most cases.

Fig. 5.8 d, e

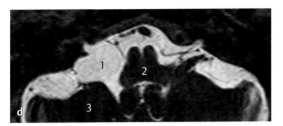

d MRI, T2-weighted, axial. Arachnoids cysts are frequently asymptomatic and noted as incidental findings on CT or MRI. They can be difficult to diagnose because of similar intensity of the cyst contents and the surrounding cerebrospinal fluid, as demonstrated in this figure on the right side (1): there is some asymmetry of the brain stem (2) and cerebellum (3) on the two sides, probably due to minor compression.

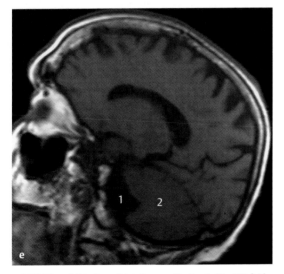

e MRI, T1-weighted, sagittal. Same patient as in **Fig. 5.8 d**. The right-sided arachnoid cyst (1) is compressing the cerebellum (2) anteriorly. The lesion does not have solid components, as is sometimes seen in schwannomas with cystic degeneration (shown elsewhere).

(Epi)dermoid Cyst

Differential Diagnosis

Arachnoid cyst, cholesterol granuloma, cystic schwannoma, vascular tumors (hemangioma, endolymphatic sac tumor). Rare: cysticercosis, dermoid and congenital cysts.

Points of Evaluation

- Epidermoid cysts can be differentiated from other pathologies, such as arachnoid cysts, with DWI. Arachnoid cysts and other water-containing cysts and tumors have low signal intensity on DWI.
- On MRI, lipomas are hyperintense on T1-weighted and hypointense on T2-weighted sequences.
- Cysticercosis is seen in endemic areas and the lesions are often smaller in size.

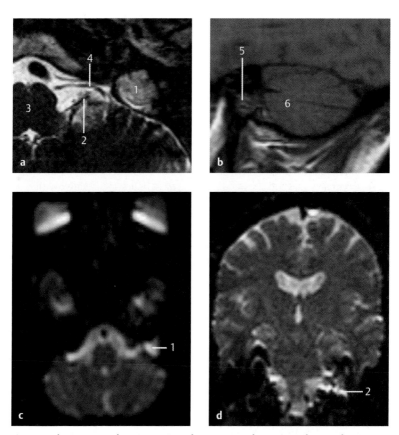

Fig. 5.9 a–d Patient with progressive and asymmetrical perceptive hearing loss.

a, b MRI, T2-weighted, axial (a) and T1-weighted, sagittal (b). MRI revealed a small fundal schwannoma in the left internal auditory canal (not shown). However, on lower slices of the T2-weighted image, a hyperintense lesion in the skull base was observed as a coincidental finding (1). Note the glossopharyngeal and/or vagal nerves (2) arising from the brainstem (3), and the anterior inferior cerebellar artery (4). On the T1-weighted image, the lesion is isointense (5) and located anterior to the cerebellum (6).

c, d Diffusion-weighted imaging. The lesion is hyperintense, as demonstrated in the axial view (1) and coronal view (2). This is typical of cholesteatoma and epidermoid cysts. Note: The bright lines on the coronal image at the border of the temporal lobe are probably an artifact.

Cholesteatoma with Intracranial Involvement

Differential Diagnosis

Lesions in the mastoid region of the skull base: congenital or acquired cholesteatoma, epidermoid and dermoid cysts, mucocele, endolymphatic sac tumor, inflammatory or autoimmune lesions, meningo(encephalo)cele, meningioma.

Points of Evaluation

- Epidermoid cysts and cholesterol granulomas are more frequently located in the petrous apex.
- Endolymphatic sac tumor originates in the region between the posterior semicircular canal and the middle cranial fossa and sigmoid sinus, with typical imaging patterns (see separate sections).
- A meningo(encephalo)cele or meningioma demonstrates osseous destruction in the middle or posterior skull base, as well as continuity with the dural or intracranial structures.

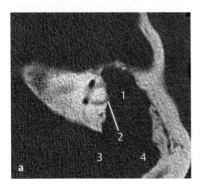

Fig. 5.10 a–g   Patient with chronic otitis media with purulent discharge.
a   CT, axial. The middle ear was fully opacified with destruction of the ossicular chain. In this slice, the opacification of the epitympanic and mastoid spaces (1) is suggestive of a mass, with erosion of the horizontal semicircular canal (2) and bony destruction toward the posterior cranial fossa (3) and sigmoid sinus (4).

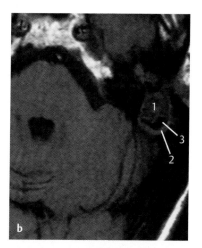

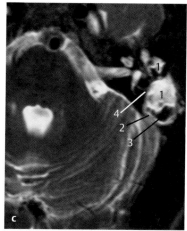

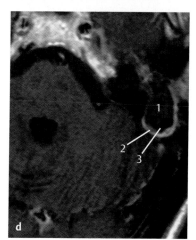

Fig. 5.10 b–d
b–d MRI, T1-weighted, (b), T2-weighted (c), and T1-weighted with gadolinium enhancement (d), axial. MRI shows better details of the characteristics and the relation of the lesion with the surrounding structures. The mass (1) is hypointense on T1-weighted and hyperintense on T2-weighted images. The capsule (2) shows gadolinium enhancement, and probably consists of highly vascularized granulation tissue due to chronic inflammation. These findings are consistent with a cholesteatoma in which the intralesional keratin shows no enhancement with gadolinium. In the posterior part of the lesion (3), some air is probably trapped, demonstrated by the lack of signal on all sequences. There is contact between the lesion and the horizontal semicircular canal (4), as seen in **Fig. 5.10a** (label 2).

Fig. 5.10 e–g ▷

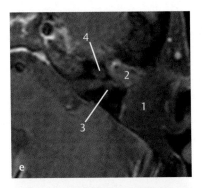

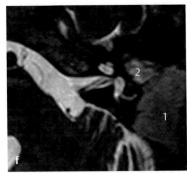

Fig. 5.10 e–g

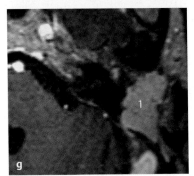

e–g MRI, T1-weighted, (e), T2-weighted (f), and T1-weighted with gadolinium enhancement (g), axial. Same patient as demonstrated on the previous figures, 5 years after surgical removal of the cholesteatoma by subtotal petrosectomy, closure of the external auditory canal, and obliteration of the cavity by abdominal fat. The abdominal fat is filling the cavity (1). Anteriorly, on the T1- and T2-weighted images, a slight hyperintense lesion (2) is observed, which may be a residual cholesteatoma. The inner ear structures with their fluid contents are best visualized on the T2-weighted image; there is partial destruction of the horizontal semicircular canal (3) but the cochlea is intact (4).

Cystic Degeneration in CPA Schwannoma

Differential Diagnosis

Arachnoid cyst, mucocele, hemangioblastoma.

Points of Evaluation

- An arachnoid cyst may be secondary to folding or inclusion of arachnoid membranes by compression from a schwannoma or meningioma. They are mostly located outside the margin of the causative lesion.
- A mucocele may be considered when the cyst is in located in a structure covered by mucosa.
- Although a hemangioblastoma only rarely presents as a CPA lesion, it may undergo rapidly progressive and massive cystic degeneration with partial enhancement of its solid parts, as is frequently observed in Von Hippel–Lindau disease.

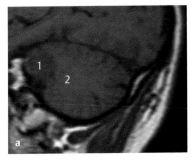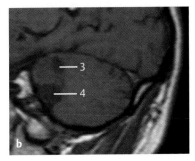

Fig. 5.11 a–d Patient with a vestibular schwannoma evaluated by a wait-and-see policy.

a, b MRI, T1-weighted, sagittal. The left image shows a schwannoma (1) of the CPA with minor compression of the cerebellum (2). In the right image, 1 year after a wait-and-watch policy, the lesion has expanded rapidly due to cystic changes in the posterior cranial (3) and caudal (4) regions, while the primary (solid) part of the schwannoma has not enlarged in size.

Fig. 5.11 c, d ▷

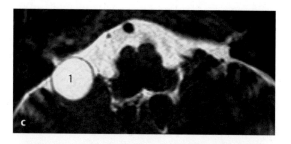

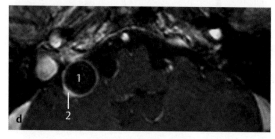

Fig. 5.11 c, d

c, d MRI, T2-weighted (c) and T1-weighted with gadolinium enhancement (d), axial. A caudal slice (left) demonstrates a round cystic lesion (1) with a thin capsule. The signal intensity is identical to the surrounding cerebrospinal fluid. No solid parts are visible at this level. To prevent misinterpreting the lesion as an arachnoid cyst, continuity of this cystic area with the solid part of the schwannoma should be established on adjacent sections. With gadolinium, the cystic part of the lesion is not enhanced (1), while in the solid parts enhancement is observed (2). Although there are therapeutic options available for rapidly expanding lesions, predicting their effect preoperatively remains difficult.

Effects of Radiotherapy on CPA Schwannoma

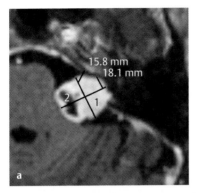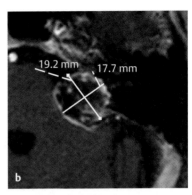

Fig. 5.12 a, b   Patient with a growing vestibular schwannoma treated with fractionated stereotactic radiotherapy.

a MRI, T1-weighted with gadolinium enhancement, axial. In an attempt to preserve residual hearing, the patient opted for fractionated stereotactic radiotherapy. Prior to treatment, a solid, enhancing tumor in the CPA (1) with a small cyst (2) was observed.

b MRI, T1-weighted with gadolinium enhancement, axial. After radiation therapy, the patient's symptoms worsened, and repeat MRI showed some enlargement and severe vacuolization of the tumor. These signs are often encountered shortly after radiotherapy, but with time, the tumor shrinks because of fibrosis. The chances of preservation of hearing are difficult to determine before treatment.

Neurofibromatosis II (NF II)

Differential Diagnosis

Multiple lesions and involvement of organs are also seen in Von Hippel–Lindau disease and inflammatory disorders such as sarcoidosis and syphilis.

Points of Evaluation

- Neurofibromatosis may initially present as otologic deficits.
- The only ENT finding in cases of Von Hippel–Lindau disease is the presence of a unilateral or bilateral endolymphatic sac tumor.
- Inflammatory diseases often have a rapidly progressive clinical course with multiple cranial nerve deficits, sometimes in combination with meningitis.

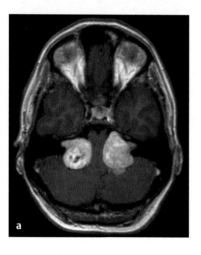

Fig. 5.13 a–f   22-year-old woman with headache, facial weakness on the right side, and sensory disturbances in the left face.
a MRI, T1-weighted with gadolinium enhancement, axial. Bilateral CPA lesions, typical of schwannoma. The left mass has an anterior extension that is compressing the trigeminal nerve. Treatment options are dependent on hearing levels and degree of compression of the brainstem between the two lesions. Radiotherapy carries a risk of initial enlargement of the radiated lesion(s) and simultaneous radiotherapy-induced edema of the brainstem. Genetic evaluation confirmed the diagnosis of NF II, without any known family history.

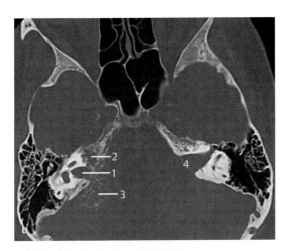

Fig. 5.13 b–f Another patient with NF II.

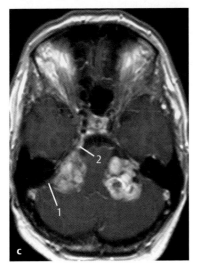

b CT, axial. Note the slight widening of the right auditory canal (1), irregular osseous destructions in the petrous apex (2), and calcifications (3) suggestive of meningioma. The left internal auditory canal is greatly distended without any irregular bony outline or calcifications (4), which is more characteristic of schwannoma.

c MRI, T1-weighted with gadolinium enhancement, axial. MRI of the same patient as in **Fig. 5.13 b**, confirming the suspicion of bilateral CPA lesions. Both tumors are multilobulated with cystic components. The right side seems to show a dural tail, is in broad contact with the dura (1) and has an anterior dural extension as demonstrated by contrast enhancement (2), suggestive of meningioma. The left tumor is somewhat more typical of a schwannoma.

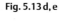

Fig. 5.13 d, e

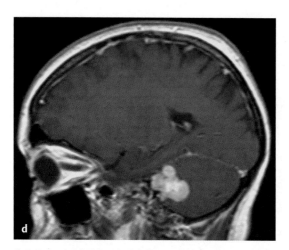

d MRI, T1-weighted with gadolinium enhancement, sagittal.
Again, this time on a sagittal view, the multilobulated mass on the left side is associated with cerebellar compression, but there is no sign of infiltration.

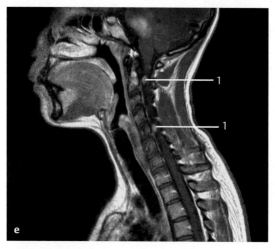

e MRI, T1-weighted with gadolinium enhancement, sagittal.
Other schwannomas in NF II may arise in the medulla (1), as shown on this thoracic slice. These lesions may in time give rise to (intra)medullar compression, with pain syndromes and a variety of neurologic deficits as a consequence. Anterior to the cerebellum, the left CPA lesion that is shown in a previous figure is visible.

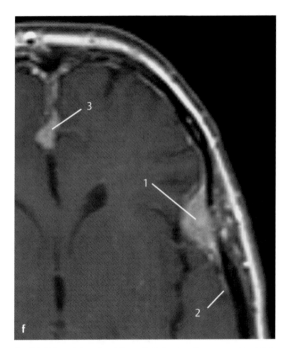

Fig. 5.13 f

f MRI, T1-weighted with gadolinium enhancement, axial.
Although in neuro-otology, scanning is focused on the CPA, lesions may be found in other intracranial sites. On this axial slice, a temporal meningioma (1) is demonstrated with a typical so-called dural tail following the dura (2). Another smaller meningioma is present adjacent to the falx cerebri (3).

Meningioma of the Cerebellopontine Angle

Differential Diagnosis
Schwannoma, pachymeningitis (in cases of smaller masses). Less likely: ependymoma, astrocytoma.

Points of Evaluation
On CT, meningioma may be associated with calcifications and hyperostosis of the surrounding bony structures. In the case below, although hearing was restored subjectively and confirmed by audiometry, brainstem audiometry revealed evidence of persisting severe retrocochlear pathology. Meningiomas originating and staying localized within the internal auditory canal are possible but extremely rare; they usually protrude into the canal from a CPA location, as shown in this case. The internal auditory canal may be enlarged due to expansion by the tumor, or narrowed due to hyperostotic changes. The presence of a dural tail is suggestive but not pathognomic of meningioma.

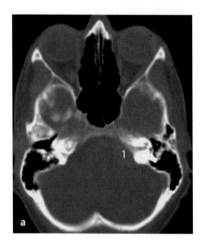

Fig. 5.14 a–c   A 35-year-old woman who developed sudden deafness on the left side and numbness on the left side of her face during pregnancy.
a CT, axial. Just before the birth of her child, screening with CT without contrast enhancement suggested a lesion in the left CPA (1). The size of the internal auditory canal does not seem to be affected. No abnormalities are noted on the right side. After birth, hearing was restored completely. Nevertheless, MRI was carried out for further evaluation.

Fig. 5.14 b, c

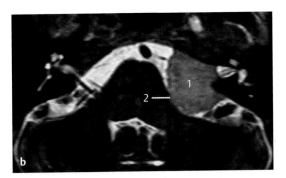

b MRI, T2-weighted, axial. MRI revealed a mass in the CPA (1) that was touching the brainstem (2) and had a significant anterior extension, with some growth into the internal auditory canal.

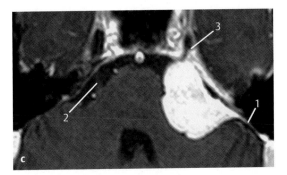

c MRI, T1-weighted with gadolinium enhancement, axial. Strong enhancement of the mass with a dural tail posteriorly (1). The sensory disturbances may be explained by the compression of the trigeminal nerve. On the contralateral healthy side, the course of the trigeminal nerve from the brainstem is indicated (2). On the affected (left) side, this area is fully invaded by tumor, with protrusion into the Meckel cave (3).

Trigeminal Nerve Schwannoma

Differential Diagnosis

Ependymoma, cholesterol granuloma (petrous apex), inflammatory disorders with gumma (sarcoidosis, syphilis).

Points of Evaluation

- Initial and later clinical symptoms are suggestive of the site of origin of the lesion as well as helping in differentiation between a tumor and inflammatory lesion.
- Multiple lesions or cranial nerve deficits and rapid progression are indicative of inflammatory disorders.

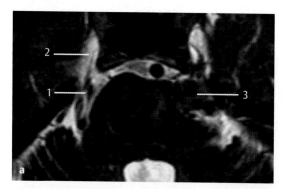

Fig. 5.15 a–d Trigeminal nerve schwannoma.

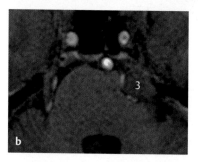

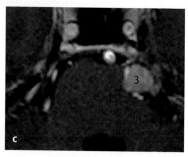

a–c Patient with left facial sensory deficits: MRI, T2-weighted (a), T1-weighted (b), and T1-weighted with gadolinium enhancement (c), axial. The T2-weighted image (left figure) shows a normal apppearance of cerebrospinal fluid surrounding (1) the root entry zone of the trigeminal nerve from the brainstem, and normal appearance of the Meckel cave on the right side (2). On the left side, a mass lesion (3) is seen at the expected position of the trigeminal nerve root entry zone. This mass has a rounded, benign appearance and is enhancing homogeneously. These imaging characteristics, in combination with the clinical symptoms, are strongly suggestive of trigeminal nerve schwannoma.

Fig. 5.15 d

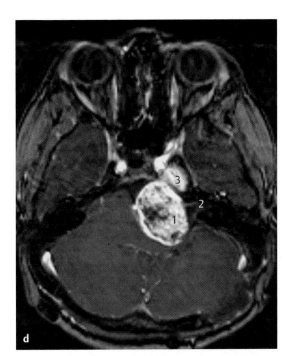

d MRI, T1-weighted with gadolinium enhancement, axial.
Sometimes the localization of the primary tumor is difficult, as demonstrated in this case with trigeminal nerve dysfunction. There is a smooth-bordered mass in the CPA. The posterior part of this mass (1), which is compressing the brainstem and cerebellum, shows nonhomogeneous contrast enhancement with severe cystic/necrotic nonenhancing areas. The internal auditory canal has a normal appearance (2). The anterior part of the mass, at the expected position of the Meckel cave (3), is enhanced homogeneously. The imaging findings are nonspecific and the differential diagnosis includes vestibulocochlear and facial schwannomas (without extension into the internal auditory canal), meningioma, and trigeminal schwannoma. The anterior extension into the Meckel cave favors the latter in combination with the clinical presentation.

Astrocytoma in the Cerebellopontine Angle

Differential Diagnosis
- Meningioma or schwannoma with cystic degeneration, malignant transformation (rare), or residual tumor after surgical debulking. Other primary brainstem lesions such as ependymoma and glioma.
- Infiltrative endolymphatic sac tumor.

Points of Evaluation
- Sharpness of the margins helps to differentiate between a benign and malignant lesion.
- An endolymphatic sac tumor originating near the osseous mastoid part behind the labyrinth is mostly confined extradurally.

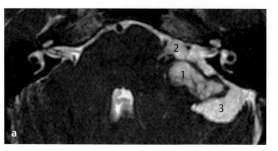

Fig. 5.16 a–c   Incidental finding of a lesion in the left posterior cranial fossa in a young female after head trauma. No hearing loss was present, although brainstem-evoked response audiometry was abnormal.

a MRI, T2-weighted, axial. A fluid-rich (1) area of heterogenous intensity was observed intradurally in the cerebellum, with doubtful extension (2) to the orifice of the internal auditory canal. A collection of cerebrospinal fluid surrounds the lesion (3).

Fig. 5.16 b, c

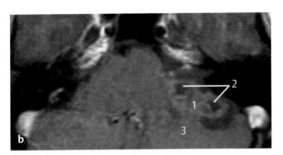

b MRI, T1-weighted with gadolinium enhancement, axial.
Note the subtle contrast enhancement. More clearly visualized
are the solid contents (1) with irregular outlines, cystic components (2), and invasion of the cerebellum (3).

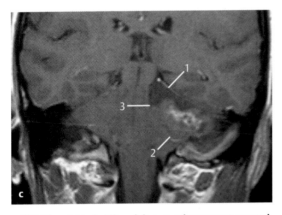

c MRI, T1-weighted with gadolinium enhancement, coronal.
The normal enhancement pattern of the tentorium is well
demonstrated on this coronal view (1) and separates the partly
enhancing cerebellar tumor from the normal supratentorial
structures. Also, the caudal (2) and medial (3) tumor margins
are better appreciated as demonstrated by the substantial extension into the left cerebellar hemisphere.

Labyrinthitis and Subclinical Meningitis

Differential Diagnosis

Most frequently viral labyrinthitis; bacterial labyrinthitis may be secondary to middle ear diseases (true bacterial invasion or because of endotoxin transport), autoimmune disorders (Cogan disease) or spread from retrocochlear pathology (see also next section on otosyphilis).

Points of Evaluation

- Otoscopy may exclude middle ear infections although CT may be indicated in some cases. MRI will show (retro)cochlear enhancement in cases of (acute) infections.
- Inflammatory involvement of the intralabyrinthine structures may result in fibrosis and ossification. In bilateral cases, this may hamper insertion of a cochlear implant.

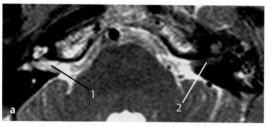

a MRI, T2-weighted, axial. Note the normal fluid content of the internal auditory canal on the right side (1), whereas on the affected side, the internal auditory canal (2) and the inner ear contents are hypointense.

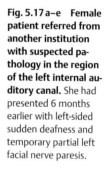

Fig. 5.17 a–e Female patient referred from another institution with suspected pathology in the region of the left internal auditory canal. She had presented 6 months earlier with left-sided sudden deafness and temporary partial left facial nerve paresis.

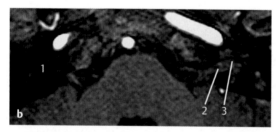

b MRI, T1-weighted, axial. Normally, as seen on the healthy side, inner ear structures are barely visible on T1-weighted images (1). However, in this patient, the left internal auditory canal contents (2) as well as the inner ear structures (3) are well visualized because of their pathologic, intermediate signal intensity.

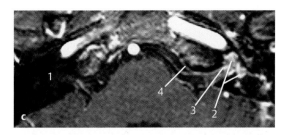

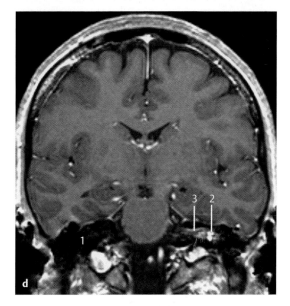

Fig. 5.17 c–e

c, d MRI, T1-weighted with gadolinium enhancement, axial (c) and coronal (d). Contrast-enhanced MRI shows no enhancement of the normal right side (1). On the left side, there is marked enhancement of the cochlea, vestibule (2) and a small part of the internal auditory canal (3). Note the subtle meningeal thickening and enhancement along the cerebellopontine cistern (4). All these findings are suggestive of labyrinthitis with intraluminal fibrosis and/or ossification, in combination with subclinical meningitis.

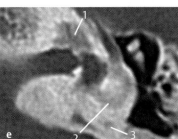

e CT axial. Further evaluation with CT confirmed the suspected ossification of the cochlea (1) and the horizontal (2) and posterior (3) semicircular canals.

Otosyphilis and Intracranial Complications

Differential Diagnosis

Pachymeningitis may be caused by:

- *Infections* other than the below described syphilis (*Treponema pallidum*): tuberculosis, Lyme disease (*Borrelia burgdorferi*), fungal, cysticercosis, T-cell lymphoma virus.
- *Autoimmune diseases* such as rheumatoid arthritis, Wegener granulomatosis, sarcoidosis, polyarteritis nodosa, Behçet disease, Sjögren disease.
- *Neoplasms* such as lymphoma, plasmacytoma, meningioma, metastasis.

Points of Evaluation

- Cranial nerve deficits, rapid progression, and multiple lesions are strongly indicative of inflammatory disorders. If malignancy is suspected, beware of involvement of other organs as primary sites of possible metastases.
- Inflammatory involvement of the intralabyrinthine structures may result in fibrosis and/or ossification. In bilateral cases, this may hamper insertion of a cochlear implant, although its success may also be restricted by retrocochlear deficits.

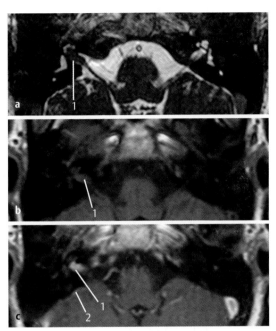

Fig. 5.18 a–f   Two weeks prior to this MRI investigation, this young man presented with sudden deafness of the right ear, followed by severe vertigo and headaches. He also had sensory disturbances in his left face and weakness in his left arm. The patient was referred after detection of a lesion in the CPA, which was classified as a vestibular schwannoma.

a–c MRI, T2-weighted (a), T1-weighted (b), and T1-weighted with gadolinium enhancement (c), axial. The T2-weighted images demonstrate absence of fluid in the internal auditory canal near the fundus (1), suggestive of schwannoma. However, on T1-weighted imaging, the lesion in the internal auditory canal (1), and also the inner ear structures have pathologic, intermediate signal intensity (compare with the normal left side). Post-gadolinium administration, there is enhancement of the internal auditory canal lesion (1) but not of the inner ear structures. In the adjacent area, there is some subtle dural enhancement along the cerebellum (2).

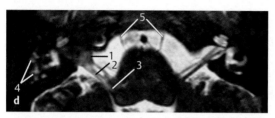

Fig. 5.18 d, e

d MRI, T2-weighted, axial. After referral, progressive partial facial paresis developed. For this reason and other persisting complaints, a second MRI was undertaken 11 days later, showing enlargement of the internal auditory canal lesion with bulging into the cerebellopontine cistern (1). The cranial nerves running through the internal auditory canal (2) are thickened along their entire course from the root entry zone in the brainstem (3). Furthermore, a few mastoid air cells around the labyrinth now contain fluid (4). Note: bilateral normal appearance of the abducens nerves (5)

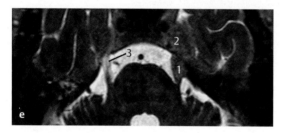

e MRI, axial, setting indicated. Retrospective examination of the initial MRI revealed a mass lesion in the left trigeminal nerve, extending from the root entry zone (1) toward the trigeminal ganglion in the Meckel cave (2). This could well explain the sensory facial disturbances on the left side. The right trigeminal nerve is normal in its course through the cerebrospinal fluid (3).

Fig. 5.18 f

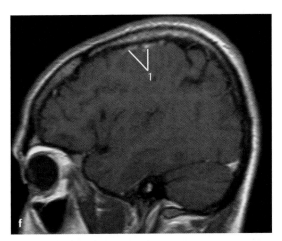

f MRI with gadolinium, sagittal. There is pachymeningeal enhancement at the convexity (1), suggestive of meningitis, which explains the severe headaches experienced by this patient. The severe headaches were explained by the meningitis, which was confirmed by the enhancement in the upper region of the temporal lobe (1). Also, the patient had sensory disturbances of the left (contralateral) face and loss of strength of the left arm. Lumbar puncture elicited a cloudy fluid with leukocytes. Serologic examination was positive for *Treponema pallidum*.

Osseous Destruction of the Temporal Bone

Endolymphatic Sac Tumor

Differential Diagnosis
Glomus jugulotympanicum, hemangioma, meningioma, middle ear tumors (adenoma, cholesteatoma), hematologic malignancies, chondrosarcoma, metastasis.

Points of Evaluation
- Endolymphatic sac tumor arising from the middle third of the endolymphatic sac. It is a hypervascular tumor that may show intratumorous calcification. Bone destruction is characteristic, especially in patients with known Von Hippel–Lindau disease.
- Remember to consider the possibility of bone destruction in the region of the jugular bulb and jugular foramen and the anticipated clinical symptoms with growth of the tumor when discussing the remaining surgical options with the patient, in particular the effects on cranial nerves VII–XI.
- An endolymphatic sac tumor is associated with a high risk of progressive morbidity and surgical complications because of excessive bleeding and cranial nerve damage. Preoperative embolization is recommended if possible.

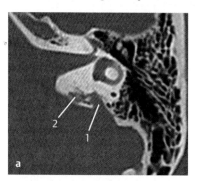 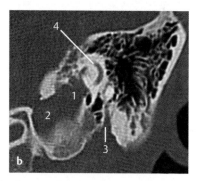

Fig. 5.19 a–e   Patient with Von Hippel–Lindau disease referred for ENT-screening.

a CT, axial. This axial view shows destruction of the posteromedial temporal bone at the expected position of the endolymphatic sac, characteristic of endolymphatic sac tumor. The vestibular aqueduct may be widened (1), and in most cases, there is invasion of the surrounding bone (2) with extension to the jugular bulb, internal auditory canal, mastoid, and inner ear structures. Intracranial involvement is evaluated better with MRI.

b CT, coronal. The largest part of the tumor (1) is on the roof of the jugular bulb (2), with some infiltration of the medial mastoid cells up to the middle cranial fossa. Note the intact stylomastoid foramen (3) and posterior semicircular canal (4). As in the present case, these tumors are more frequently found in patients with **Von Hippel–Lindau disease**. Apart from this, endolymphatic sac tumor is a rare entity.

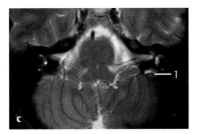

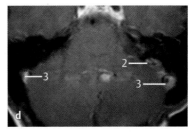

Fig. 5.19 c–e

c MRI, T2-weighted, axial. The tumor is visible as an area of increased signal intensity in the posteromedial part of the temporal bone (1), just posterior to the normal fluid signal of the posterior semicircular canal, confirming the CT findings.

d MRI, T1-weighted with gadolinium enhancement, axial. Post-contrast imaging shows strong enhancement of the lesion on the left side (2), confirming its hypervascularity, as well as the normal flow in the sigmoid sinus on both sides (3).

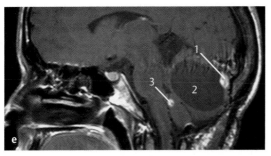

e MRI, T1-weighted with gadolinium enhancement, sagittal. Patients with Von Hippel–Lindau disease can have several other tumors associated with marked morbidity because of compression of vital structures and secondary hydrocephalus. In this case, **hemangioblastoma**, with an enhancing solid (1) and a nonenhancing large cystic (2) component is severely compressing the cerebellum. A secondary, small enhancing tumor is seen more anteriorly (3).

Glomus Jugulare Tumor (Paraganglioma)

Differential Diagnosis
Glomus tympanicum, hemangioma, middle ear tumors (adenoma, cholesteatoma), hematologic malignancies, metastasis.

Points of Evaluation
The hypotympanic floor may also be eroded by inferior growth of a glomus tympanicum tumor. Erosion of the cortical outline of the jugular fossa, the hypotympanic floor, and the bony canal of the carotid artery on CT, as well as heterogeneous intensities, flow voids, and concomitant compression or obstruction of the flow in the jugular bulb on MRI, are highly suggestive of glomus jugulare or glomus jugulotympanicum tumor.

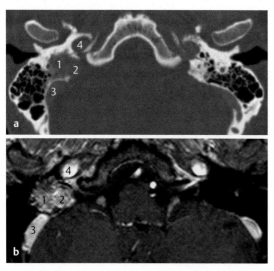

Fig. 5.20 a–c Patient with pulsating tinnitus, without any pathology behind the eardrum.

a, b CT and MRI, T1-weighted with gadolinium enhancement, axial. CT shows moth-eaten bone destruction of the jugular foramen, characteristic of a jugular paraganglioma. The post-gadolinium MR image shows strong, slightly nonhomogeneous, enhancement of the paraganglioma (1); the area of the jugular bulb also seems to be involved (2), with some areas of signal void representing intratumoral vessels (so-called salt and pepper pattern). The sigmoid sinus (3) and internal carotid artery (4) are not affected.

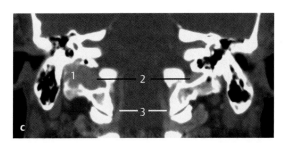

Fig. 5.20 c

c CT with intravenous contrast enhancement, coronal. Enhancing mass (1) with bone destruction in and around the right jugular foramen, which is widened compared with the normal left side (2). There is normal enhancement of the carotid arteries or vertebral arteries bilaterally (3). Note that the floor of the tympanic cavity is intact, which makes the lesion a true glomus jugulare tumor. If this type of lesion grows through the inferior wall of the tympanic cavity, it should be classified as a glomus jugulotympanicum.

Lymphangioma

Differential Diagnosis
Pseudotumors, mucocele, cholesterol cyst (granuloma); less likely due to its contents: hemangioma, cholesteatoma, epidermoid cysts, and arachnoid cyst of the petrous apex.

Points of Evaluation
- Presence of septations (as seen in this patient) in the lesion favors lymphangioma.
- Pseudotumors of the petrous apex are often incidental findings (see separate section).
- Hemangioma has a salt and pepper configuration, although it is very rare in the petrous apex.
- A cholesterol cyst (granuloma) is hyperintense on T2-weighted sequences due to mucus stasis, and hyperintense on T1-weighted sequences due to hemorrhagic changes, with possible contrast enhancement of the capsule and expansive characteristics.
- Cholesteatoma is less bright on T1-weighted sequences.
- Epidermoid cysts demonstrate hypointense T1-weighted and hyperintense T2-weighted signals.

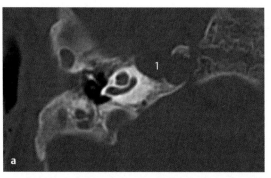

Fig. 5.21 a–c Young male patient presenting with repeated episodes of meningitis of unknown cause.

a CT, axial. In the petrous apex, a smooth-bordered, expanding lesion (1) has destroyed some bony cells in the apex, as well as part of the otic capsule. The cochlear lumen is intact. Some mastoid cells are visible and opacified.

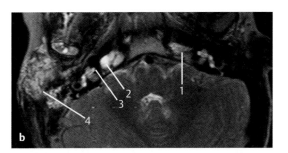

Fig. 5.21 b, c

b MRI, T2-weighted, axial. MRI shows the differences between the opacities much more clearly than the CT scan. In the left petrous apex, the fatty bone marrow is hyperintense (1). The lesion visible on CT has a uniform high signal intensity (2), identical to the normal fluid present in the cochlea (3), vestibule, and semicircular canals. This confirms the cystic nature of this expanding lesion. Anteriorly, as on other slices, due to compression of the eustachian tube stasis of mucosal secretions in the mastoid is seen (4).

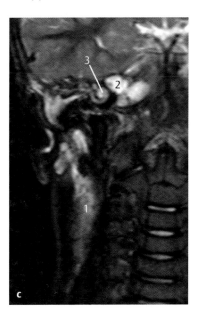

c MRI, T2-weighted, coronal. Most lymphangiomas are found in the neck, as is the case in our patient, who has extensive spread of lymphangioma on the right side of his neck (1). In some patients, lymphangioma may not only spread throughout the neck structures but also expand rapidly with complications because of compression of vital structures. The lesion (2), as demonstrated in the previous figures, is separated from the intracochlear lumen (3).

Infection of the Skull Base and Gradenigo Syndrome

Differential Diagnosis

- Common infections spreading from the middle ear and mastoid.
- Infections affecting multiple cranial nerves (see section on otosyphilis above).
- Solitary tumors of the trigeminal or abducens nerve.
- Concomitant compression by skull base tumors (schwannoma, meningioma, dermoid, chordoma, chondrosarcoma).

Points of Evaluation

- In Gradenigo syndrome, the dural branches of the first division of the trigeminal nerve are involved in the symptoms of pain; the abducens nerve is paralyzed because of compression in the Dorello canal in the petrous apex. Pseudo-Gradenigo may be due to a nasopharyngeal carcinoma infiltrating the skull base.
- Malignant otitis externa may lead to skull-base infection. Immunocompromised and diabetic patients are prone to bacterial (e.g., *Pseudomonas*) or fungal (e.g., *Aspergillus*) infections. Sequential radiographic and radionuclide (e. g., technetium and gallium) imaging may be used to monitor the efficacy of treatment. Complications may result from the spread of infection to adjacent intracranial or head and neck structures.

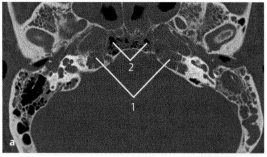

a CT, axial. The petrous apex on both sides (1) is opacified. This could be because of normal fatty marrow but, considering the opacification in the mastoid and the clinical symptoms, is more suggestive of trapped fluid within the pneumatized apices. Also, the clivus contains multiple air bubbles (2), which is grossly abnormal. These imaging findings are consistent with the presence of a necrotizing (probably bacterial) infection of the skull base with primary or secondary involvement of the temporal bones.

Fig. 5.22 a–c Patient with purulent discharge of the left ear, headaches, signs of meningitis, and diplopia because of unilateral dysfunction of the left abducens nerve, all classic features of Gradenigo syndrome.

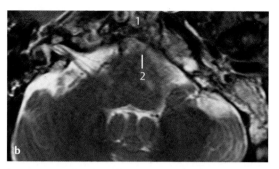

Fig. 5.22 b, c

b MRI, T2-weighted, axial. Opacification of the entire left and part of the right mastoids without bone destruction is confirmed. The mastoid is hyperintense comparable with the cerebrospinal fluid. The petrous apices show a somewhat intermediate signal intensity similar to that of the clivus (1). On this section, the left abducens nerve is well visualized in its course from the brainstem (2) to the area of abnormal intermediate signal intensity (the patient is positioned slightly out of the axial plane; therefore the right abducens nerve is not visible).

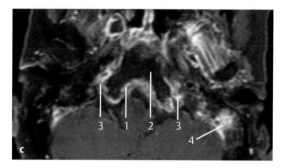

c MRI, T1-weighted with gadolinium enhancement, axial. There is abnormal enhancement of the contours of the clivus (1) with central hypointensity (probably necrosis) and air bubbles (2). Also, the petrous apices are enhanced (3). Note the trapped fluid in the left mastoid is also showing enhancement (4). The imaging findings are indicative of a widespread infectious process.

Petrositis

Differential Diagnosis
Pseudotumors, cystic lesions (cholesterol granuloma, mucocele, epidermoid), solid tumors (chordoma, chondroma, chondrosarcoma, giant cell tumor, metastases), endolymphatic sac tumors.

Points of Evaluation
Clinical symptoms may help differentiate between inflammatory disorders, asymptomatic pseudotumors, and other pathology. CT and MRI are complementary. Knowing whether the origin is intradural or extradural and the presence of bony changes help to establish the most likely diagnosis.

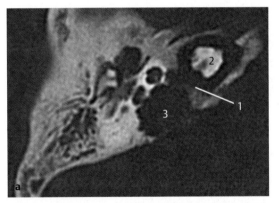

Fig. 5.23 a–c   Child with a chronic purulent otitis with complete opacification of the mastoid and middle ear. This otitis was present for many years with neglected deafness in the right ear.

a CT, axial. The internal auditory canal is seen (1), but is not clearly recognizable. Anteriorly, a rounded lucency in the petrous apex is visible with a central bone sequester (2). Posteriorly, a second area of irregular bone lysis (3) is located immediately posterior to the vestibule and cochlea.

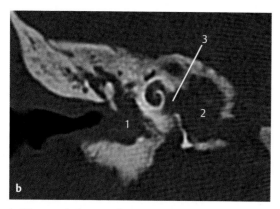

Fig. 5.23 b–c

b CT, coronal. This view shows opacification of the middle ear (1) and the expansile lytic lesion seen in **Fig. 5.23 a** anterior to the internal auditory canal (2), with destruction of the otic capsule (3) as the reason for the deafness.

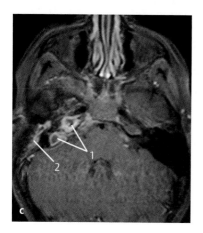

c MRI, T1-weighted with gadolinium enhancement, axial. Anterior and posterior to the internal auditory canal (1), rounded lesions are present with rim enhancement and central hypointensity suggestive of capsule formation or granulation around areas of necrosis. The adjacent dura shows reactive thickening and increased enhancement. Also, some enhancement is seen in the trapped fluid in the mastoid (2), indicative of chronic otitis. The clinical symptoms and imaging findings together lead to a diagnosis of chronic granulomatous infection with capsule formation in and around the inner ear and petrous apex, causing extensive bone destruction with deafness as a result.

Fibrous Dysplasia of the Skull Base

Differential Diagnosis

Paget disease, osteopetrosis (Albers–Schönberg), craniometaphyseal dysplasia, McCune–Albright syndrome.

Points of Evaluation

- In later stages of Paget disease, the otic capsule is completely resorbed. Osteopetrosis demonstrates a complete lack of pneumatization of the temporal bone. Craniometaphyseal dysplasia is recognized by the presence of increased bone densities.
- Beware of encroachment of vital structures and cranial nerves as well as the formation of an inclusion cholesteatoma.

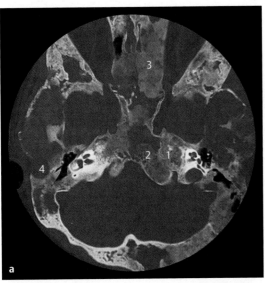

Fig. 5.24 a, b Patients with McCune–Albright syndrome complaining of subcutaneous bony swelling and hearing loss.

a CT, axial. All visualized bones are enlarged with a dense "ground glass" appearance and intact cortical outlines. These imaging findings are characteristic of polyostotic fibrous dysplasia. The petrous apex (1) and clivus (2) are hardly recognizable and there is severe deformity of the anterior skull base in the area of the cribriform plate (3). The deformities may cause narrowing of the skull base foramina resulting in progressive compression and paralysis of multiple cranial nerves. Another consequence may be stenosis of the external auditory canal, risk of inclusion cholesteatoma (4), and deformities of the middle ear, resulting in conductive hearing loss.

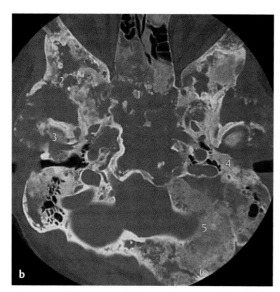

Fig. 5.24 b

b CT, axial. The deformities in the anterior skull base (1), resulting in anosmia, are clearly visible. Also, the middle cranial fossa and infratemporal fossa are involved (2). The temporomandibular joint is hardly recognizable (3) and there are associated functional problems. On the left side, the external auditory canal is stenosed (4). In the posterior cranial fossa (5), less space is available for the cerebellum. The bulging growth pattern of the outer skull (6) may lead to cosmetic deformities.

Pathology in the Anterior Skull Base

Meningioma with Skull Base Destruction

Differential Diagnosis
- Bone dystrophies, e.g., fibrous dysplasia.
- Tumors of the paranasal sinuses, e.g., squamous cell carcinoma, angiofibroma, ossifying fibroma, chordoma, eosinophilic granuloma.
- Very rare: malignant degenerated schwannoma.

Points of Evaluation
- On CT, the bone changes associated with hyperostosing meningioma en plaque may be confused with (polyostotic) fibrous dysplasia. However, in meningioma the cortical margins of the affected bones are not well delineated.
- In fibrous dysplasia, the cortical margins are preserved (compare with section on fibrous dysplasia). Cranial nerves and intracranial vasculature may be encroached on by the lesion. Total surgical removal is rarely possible.

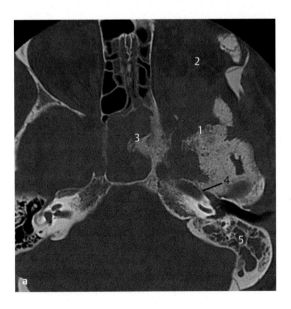

Fig. 5.25 a, b Patient with proptosis and blindness of the left eye.

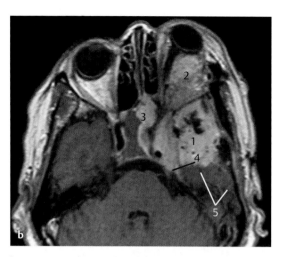

Fig. 5.25 b

b MRI, T1-weighted with gadolinium enhancement. The full extent of the meningioma can be appreciated with the areas of hyperostosis on the bone window CT showing strong enhancement (1). Enhancing tumor tissue is also present in the orbit (2) and the sphenocavernous region (3). The left proptosis and resulting displacement and stretching of the optic nerve is the cause of the patient's blindness. The cavernous sinus is invaded with tumor displacing and surrounding the internal carotid artery. Posteriorly, a dural tail sign is present (4). The retained secretions in the mastoid are not enhanced (5).

a CT, axial bone window. On the left side, osseous changes are observed in the area of the anterior fossa (1), orbit (2), and sphenoid sinus (3). The bones have remodeled and expanded because of hyperostosis. Note that the cortical margins of the involved bones are not well delineated. The eustachian tube is narrowed due to compression and infiltration by the lesion (4), resulting in stasis of mucous secretions in the middle ear and mastoid (5). These findings are characteristic of a so-called "hyperostosing meningioma en plaque."

Mucocele of the Frontal Recess

Differential Diagnosis
Meningoencephalocele, benign or malign tumors of the paranasal sinuses, schwannoma or glioma from the orbit, intracranial tumors (e.g., small esthesio-neuroblastoma).

Points of Evaluation
- Beware of large osseous lesions of the skull base, removal of which may result in protrusion of intracranial contents or marsupialization of the mucocele.
- In meningo(encephalo)cele or intracranial tumors, persistent leakage of cerebrospinal fluid may occur at biopsy.

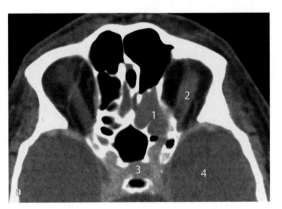

Fig. 5.26 a–c   Patient with frontal pressure and slight proptosis of the left eye.

a CT with intravenous contrast enhancement, axial. The lesion in the anterior skull base (1) in the area of the frontal recess shows signs of expansion. The cortical margins are intact. Related areas are the orbit with the superior rectus (2) with the optic nerve underneath and, more posteriorly, the pituitary gland (3). The contents of the lesion are slightly hyperdense compared with brain tissue (4).

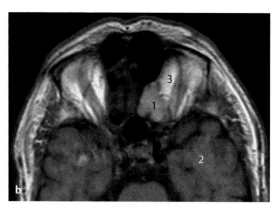

Fig. 5.26 b, c
b MRI, T1-weighted, axial. The lobulated, smooth-bordered lesion (1) at the same level as demonstrated on the CT, is suggestive of a mucocele in the frontal recess. Its hyperintense signal on the nonenhanced T1-weighted image indicates protein-rich fluid content (see Chapter 1).

Note the intermediate signal intensity of the normal brain tissue (2) and the high signal intensity of the intraorbital fat (3).

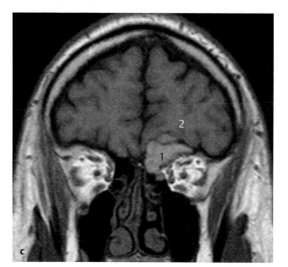

c MRI, T1-weighted, coronal. The lesion (1) is situated in the frontal recess with some extension toward the frontal sinus. The margins can be well appreciated due to the difference in signal intensity of the mucocele compared with brain tissue (2) and intraorbital fat.

Note the slight remodeling of the left orbital roof, indicative of a slow-growing lesion. Marsupialization would be an adequate treatment option in this patient, preferably with an endonasal approach.

Meningoencephalocele

Differential Diagnosis

Inclusion cysts (mucocele, epidermoid, dermoid), neoplasms (meningioma, chordoma), pituitary gland tumors. Less likely, mucocele of the lacrimal sac and duct.

Points of Evaluation

- Evaluation of the bony outlines is essential to differentiate between the sites of origin.
- Meningoencephaloceles in the lateral skull base are sometimes difficult to differentiate from (residual) cholesteatoma or facial schwannoma.

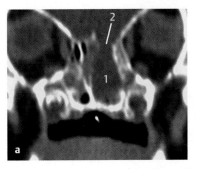 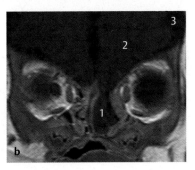

Fig. 5.27 a–c   Neonate with dyspnea and left nasal obstruction.

a CT, coronal. The left nasal cavity is filled with a soft-tissue mass (1) that seems to be connected to brain through a defect in the roof of the ethmoid (2).

b MRI, T1-weighted, coronal. This T1-weighted image confirms the CT findings. To further characterize the mass (1) it is important to observe the signal intensity. In this case, the signal intensity of the mass is similar to brain tissue (2), which fits the description a true encephalocele. If the signal intensity had been equal to that of cerebrospinal fluid (3), this would have been diagnostic of a meningocele.

Fig. 5.27 c

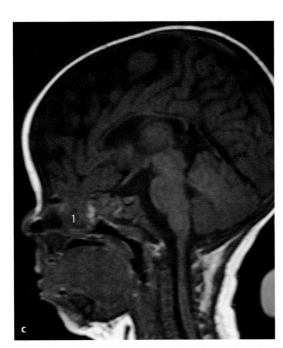

c MRI, T1-weighted, sagittal. The sagittal view confirms prolapse of the frontal lobe into the nasal cavity (1). Alternatively, repositioning could be accomplished by craniotomy and covering the skull-base defect with a muscle transplant from the inside.

Esthesioneuroblastoma

Differential Diagnosis
Meningoencephalocele, benign and malignant tumors of the paranasal sinuses (lymphoma, sarcoma, undifferentiated carcinoma), intracranial tumors.

Points of Evaluation
Esthesioneuroblastoma is an uncommon tumor of neural crest origin that arises from the olfactory mucosa in the superior nasal cavity. These polypoid tumors typically start unilaterally and may bleed profusely on biopsy. Neglected cases appear as a bilateral mass in the anterior cranial fossa. In these larger tumors, which usually have intracranial extension, peripheral tumoral cysts can occur at the margins of the intracranial part of the mass. These cysts have their broadest base on the tumor and, when present, are highly suggestive of the (imaging) diagnosis of esthesioneuroblastoma. Beware of encroachment of cranial nerves or intracranial vessels, which may be important in the estimation of morbidity during removal.

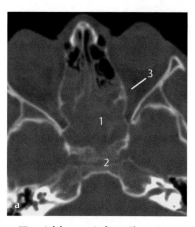

Fig. 5.28 a, b   Child with rapidly progressive bilateral nasal obstruction.

a CT, axial bone window. There is complete bilateral opacification of the ethmoid and sphenoid sinuses (1). The anterior cortex of the clivus (2) seems to be eroded, and there is some soft tissue, possibly tumor, in the left orbit (3), which is difficult to appreciate on a bone window CT image.

Fig. 5.28 b

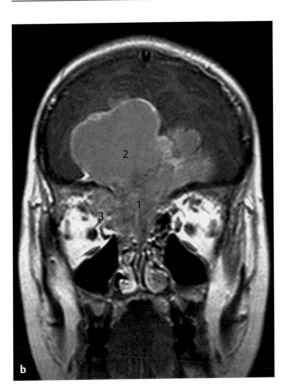

b MRI, T1-weighted with gadolinium enhancement, coronal.
A large multilobulated mass is present in the central skull base centered in the region of the cribriform plate (1) with extension bilaterally into the nasal cavity, as well as bilateral intracranial involvement. The mass shows strong enhancement possibly with a large cystic component (2) filled with high-intensity protein-rich fluid and compressing the frontal lobe. At this level, the tumor is invading the right orbital fat (3). Based on the imaging findings, esthesioneuroblastoma (olfactory neuroblastoma) is the most likely diagnosis.

Pituitary Gland Pathology

Differential Diagnosis
Meningo(encephalo)cele, mucocele, hemangioblastoma.

Points of Evaluation
- In classifications of pituitary gland pathology, lesions within the sella are classified as microadenomas. Microadenomas are frequently active hormone-producing tumors with specific clinical symptoms (e.g., galactorrhea).
- Tumors extending out of the sella are classified as macroadenomas. Most macroadenomas are nonfunctional tumors. Therefore, these lesions present late and can reach remarkable volumes. Large pituitary adenomas may be accompanied by cystic degeneration with or without hemorrhage. Macroadenomas with superior extension may compromise the optic chiasm with visual field disturbances and even blindness. Less frequently, macroadenomas spread inferiorly into the sphenoid sinus.
- Beware of large osseous lesions of the skull base, removal of which may result in protrusion of intracranial contents or marsupialization of the mucocele. In meningo(encephalo)cele or intracranial tumors, persisting leakage of cerebrospinal fluid may occur at biopsy. A trans-septal approach is a gentle approach for biopsy or surgical removal with good visualization and low risk of complications.

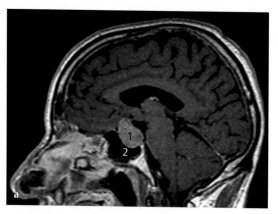

Fig. 5.29a–c Pituitary gland pathologies. The otolaryngologist may need to be consulted to provide the surgical approach for the neurosurgeon to remove the tumor.

a MRI, T1-weighted with gadolinium enhancement, sagittal. This sagittal contrast-enhanced image shows a strongly enhancing **macroadenoma** that fills the fossa sellae (1). The sella is enlarged without destruction and is extending into the roof of the sphenoid sinus (2), indicative of a slow-growing process. Superiorly it is extending to the expected position of the optic chiasm.

Fig. 5.29 b, c

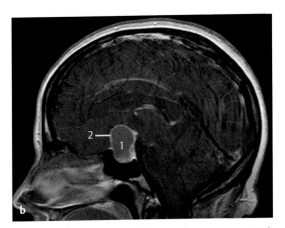

b MRI, T1-weighted with gadolinium enhancement, sagittal. Cystic pituitary gland adenoma (1), with rim enhancement (2) and suprasellar extension. Using a trans-septal or endoscopic trans-sphenoidal approach, these tumors can be resected completely or partially to resolve compression of vital structures such as the optic chiasm.

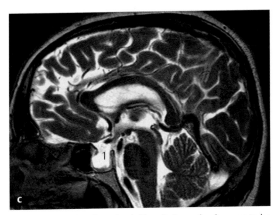

c MRI, T2-weighted, sagittal. The pituitary gland seems to be absent with the sella filled with cerebrospinal fluid (1). This is a classic case of the so-called "**empty sella**," which is usually an incidental finding of no clinical significance. The gland is flattened by compression of cerebrospinal fluid (that has herniated through the sellar diaphragm) and is visible as a thin rim of tissue along the sellar floor. The only differential diagnosis is an arachnoid cyst in the superior portion of the sella turcica.

Intracranial Complications

Dural Sinus Thrombosis

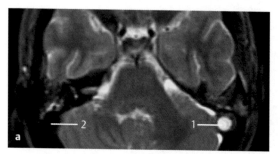

Fig. 5.30 a, b   Patient with purulent otorrhea of the left ear, fever, and severe headaches.
For evaluation, MRI with magnetic resonance angiography (MRA) is the best investigation for diagnosis of dural sinus thrombosis.

a MRI, T2-weighted, axial. Otomastoiditis can spread intracranially, resulting in dural sinus thrombophlebitis, which may compromise the sigmoid and transverse sinus and can extend into the jugular bulb or vein. This T2-weighted image shows abnormal high signal in the left sigmoid sinus (1) indicative of thrombosis. The normal right sinus (2) is patent and therefore shows no signal (so-called "flow void"). Retained secretions are present in the mastoid cells on both sides.

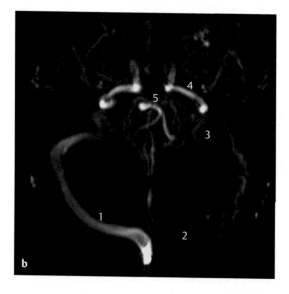

Intracranial Abscess from an Otologic Focus

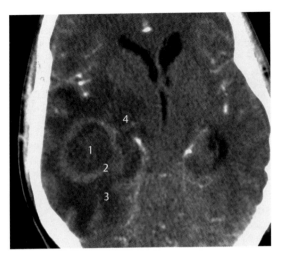

Fig. 5.31 Young male patient with a chronically infected radical cavity with a residual cholesteatoma.

CT with intravenous contrast, axial. Otomastoiditis may spread intracranially resulting in meningitis, encephalitis, and/or brain abscess. The CT image shows a right temporal abscess (1) with typical rim enhancement (2). Around the abscess, there is a large low-density area (3), indicative of brain edema with mass effect on the posterior horn of the right lateral brain ventricle (4), which is completely compressed. Unfortunately, this turned out to be a fatal complication.

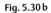
Fig. 5.30 b
b MRA, axial. The right transverse sinus is normal in appearance and patent (1). On the left side, there is complete dural thrombosis of the transverse sinus (2) and sigmoid sinus extending into the jugular bulb (3). Note the normal appearance of the internal carotid artery (4) and the basilar artery (5).

Intracranial Abscess from a Sinonasal Focus

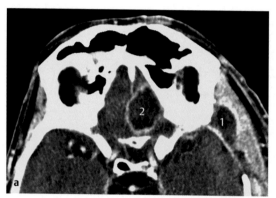

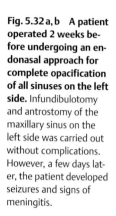

Fig. 5.32 a, b   **A patient operated 2 weeks before undergoing an endonasal approach for complete opacification of all sinuses on the left side.** Infundibulotomy and antrostomy of the maxillary sinus on the left side was carried out without complications. However, a few days later, the patient developed seizures and signs of meningitis.

a CT with intravenous contrast, axial. After initial antibiotic therapy, a subdural empyema (1) was drained surgically. In the basal left frontal lobe, a low-density area with rim enhancement is present, indicative of an intracranial abscess (2).

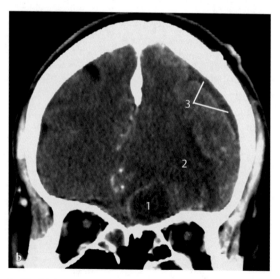

b CT with intravenous contrast, coronal. This view shows the abscess (1) in the left frontal lobe abutting the ethmoid roof. Note the extensive low-density edema (2) surrounding the abscess, and subdural fluid collection (3). After surgical drainage and antibiotics for several months, the patient recovered.

Intracranial Hemorrhage Due to a Via Falsa

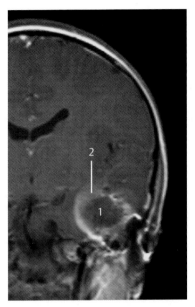

Fig. 5.33 Via falsa in a patient after an attempted mastoidectomy. The surgeon "took the wrong way" in the temporal lobe.

MRI, T1-weighted with gadolinium enhancement. The hematoma (1) has hypointense content, indicating its recent development (see Chapter 1), and there is enhancement of its margins (2). There are no signs of compression or surrounding edema.

Intracranial Hemorrhage due to a Middle Cranial Fossa Approach

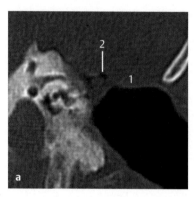 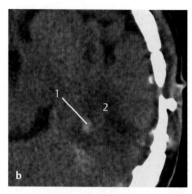

Fig. 5.34 a, b   Patient with a radical cavity and persistent loss of fluid from the cavity. The fluid proved to be cerebrospinal fluid.

a CT, coronal. The coronal image displays the radical cavity. A large bone defect is present in the expected position of the tegmen (1). Just cranial to this defect, there are some air bubbles (2), which may be located within the dura. To resolve the cerebrospinal fluid leak, the neurosurgeon opted for a middle cranial fossa approach to reconstruct the defect from the inside, supporting it with a muscle transplant.

b CT, axial. Postoperatively, the patient developed aphasia. The nonenhanced CT shows a small area of high density (1), probably fresh blood, with a large zone of surrounding edema (2). These imaging findings explain the clinical symptoms, which were probably caused by prolonged retraction of the temporal lobe during surgery.

Dural Defect after Sinonasal Surgery

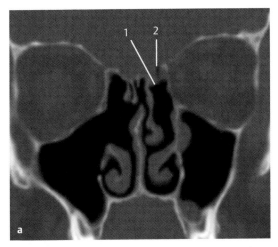

Fig. 5.35 a, b Situation after endonasal sinonasal surgery with persistent loss of cerebrospinal fluid.

a CT, coronal. This slice at the level of the olfactory fossa shows a bone defect involving the left cribriform plate (1), indicating the location of the iatrogenic cerebrospinal fluid fistula. Note the small air bubble (2) above the cribriform plate.

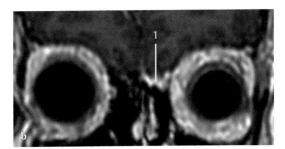

b T1-weighted MRI with gadolinium, coronal. On this T1-weighted image with gadolinium, there is strong enhancement in the region of the cerebrospinal fluid fistula (1). This is probably due to hypervascular granulation tissue and/or local meningitis.

Nose

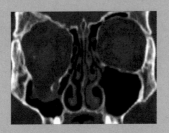

6 Radiologic Anatomy of the Nasal Cavity and Paranasal Sinuses

Conventional radiography (plain film) of the paranasal system and other parts of the skull is frequently used as a screening tool in the diagnosis of sinusitis, but has limited value for detailed evaluation due to superimposition of structures.

For more accurate preoperative evaluation and use during surgery, computed tomography (CT) is the preferred tool to visualize anatomic borders and to detect pathology in the paranasal system. Although CT does not always clearly differentiate between soft-tissue processes and secretions, it provides crucial information about disease localization and integrity of the osseous structures.

Magnetic resonance imaging (MRI) enables better discernment of the characteristics of soft-tissue disease and the relation to other anatomic structures, as well as spread to and invasion into these structures. Detailed information is provided about the intracranial compartments as well as the intraorbital structures. Examples of MRI are shown and discussed in Chapter 5.

In conventional radiography, the Caldwell view and Waters view are the most commonly used projections; these are complementary to each other.

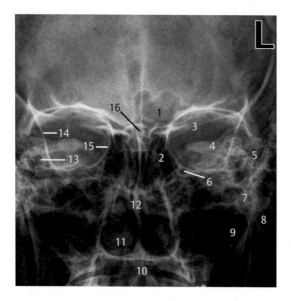

Fig. 6.1 Caldwell view
1 Left frontal sinus, right side aplasia
2 Ethmoid sinus
3 Planum sphenoidale
4 Superior aspect of the petrous bone
5 Pneumatized and aerated mastoid cells
6 Foramen rotundum (infraorbital canal)
7 Zygomatic arch (better seen on Waters view)
8 Mastoid apex
9 Maxillary sinus
10 Maxilla
11 Inferior turbinate
12 Nasal septum
13 Cochlea
14 Innominate line of the greater wing of the sphenoid
15 Lamina papyracea
16 Crista galli

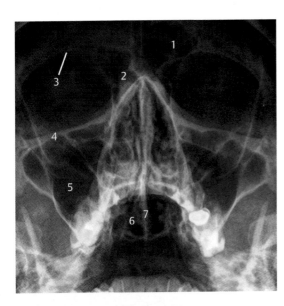

Fig. 6.2 Waters view
1 Frontal sinus
2 Frontal recess
3 Supraorbital nerve canal
4 Orbital floor
5 Maxillary sinus
6 Sphenoid sinus
7 Intersphenoidal septum

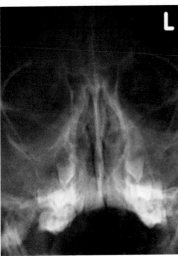

Fig. 6.3 Waters view. Waters view of a 7-year-old child. The frontal sinuses are not yet pneumatized. In the region of the maxillary sinus, several unerupted teeth are present, which limit the surgical procedures that can be carried out in this area.

Evaluation Points for CT of the Nasal Cavity and Paranasal Sinuses

Although most of the below-mentioned points of evaluation might also be evaluated on plain films, CT will demonstrate much more detail on bony outlines and contents. Systematic evaluation is best done in an anteroposterior sequence, starting with the coronal slices followed by a craniocaudal sequence of axial slices. In both sequences, the evaluation starts with the less complex slices. The paranasal sinuses as well as the remaining structures are systematically and bilaterally screened according to the points mentioned below. Although a clinical description will end up being longer, it is always worth looking at both sides in the evaluation, even in cases without pathology.

Frontal Sinus

- Presence, extension, and degree of pneumatization, bony outlines.
- Contents: septal structures, aeration or opacification of the sinus.
- In case of opacification: characteristics such as calcifications.
- Frontal recess: patency and opacification.

Ethmoid Sinus

- Degree of pneumatization, bony outlines.
- Opacification: diffuse, localization (anterior/posterior).
- Ethmoid roof: appearance, height, and left/right differences.
- Ethmoid bulla: morphology, degree of caudal extension.
- Lamina papyracea.

Infundibulum

- Patency, morphology of the uncinate process.
- Obstruction by a caudally extended ethmoid bulla, opacities.

Maxillary Sinus

- Degree of pneumatization, bony outlines, tooth elements, any fistulas from the maxilla.
- Morphology of the bony canal containing the infraorbital nerve.
- Presence of retention cysts and their relation to the natural ostium, degree of obstruction, opacifications and their characteristics.

Sphenoid Sinus

- Degree of pneumatization, bony outlines, opacification.
- Optic and internal carotid canals, foramen rotundum, pituitary fossa.

Remaining structures

- Nasal septum: deviations, septal spine or spur, crista galli.
- Nasal turbinates: morphology, pneumatization, obstructive effects.
- Cribriform plate, skull-base height differences, lacrimal duct, intraorbital pathology.

Radiologic Anatomy on Coronal CT Slices in an Anteroposterior Sequence

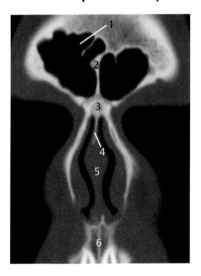

Fig. 6.4   Coronal CT slice through the sinonasal region.
1 Frontal sinus
2 Interfrontal septum
3 Os nasale/nasion
4 Perpendicular plate
5 Septal cartilage
6 Maxilla

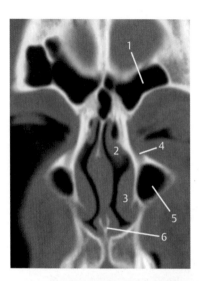

Fig. 6.5   Coronal CT slice through the sinonasal region.
1 Frontal sinus
2 Middle turbinate
3 Inferior turbinate
4 Lacrimal sac
5 Maxillary sinus
6 Anterior nasal spine

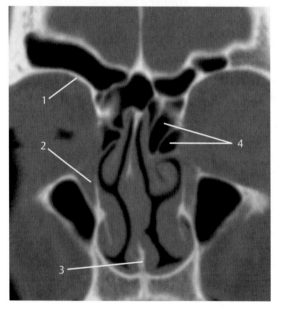

Fig. 6.6   Coronal CT slice through the sinonasal region.
1 Superior orbital margin
2 Nasolacrimal duct
3 Premaxilla
4 Anterior ethmoid cells and/or agger nasi cell (located anteriorly to the uncinate process)

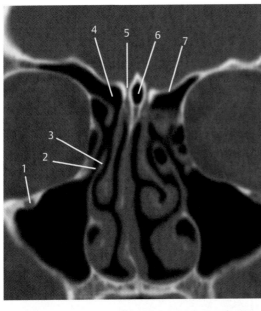

Fig. 6.7 Coronal CT slice through the sinonasal region.

1 Bony canal containing the infraorbital nerve
2 Infundibulum
3 Uncinate process (pneumatized on the left side)
4 Frontal recess
5 Cribriform plate
6 Crista galli (in this case pneumatized)
7 Fovea ethmoidalis

Note: As the point of evaluation is near the infraorbital canal, no Haller cells (infraorbital cells) are present in this case.

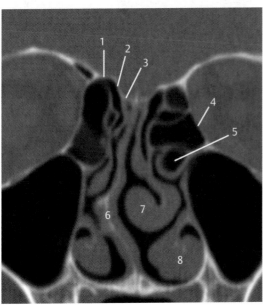

Fig. 6.8 Coronal CT slice through the sinonasal region.

1 Fovea ethmoidalis
2 Lateral lamella of the cribriform plate
3 Cribriform plate (region of cranial nerve I)
4 Lamina papyracea
5 Ethmoid bulla
6 Septal deviation with septal spur
7 Paradoxically curved middle turbinate
8 Hypertrophic inferior turbinate (might be compensatory)

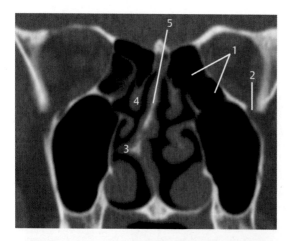

Fig. 6.9 Coronal CT slice through the sinonasal region.

1 Posterior ethmoid cells
2 Infraorbital fissure
3 Septal spine
4 Superior turbinate
5 Perpendicular plate

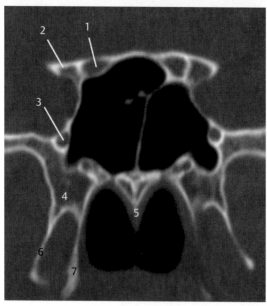

Fig. 6.10 Coronal CT slice through the sinonasal region.

1 Optic canal (cranial nerve II)
2 Anterior clinoid process
3 Foramen rotundum (cranial nerve V2, maxillary branch)
4 Pterygoid process (just behind pterygopalatine fossa, see axial slices)
5 Vomer, between the right and left choanal openings
6 Lateral lamina
7 Medial lamina

Note: In this region Onodi cells (high sphenoethmoidal cell) might be present but are not seen in this case.

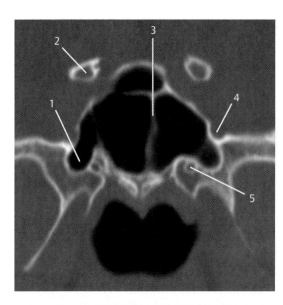

Fig. 6.11 Coronal CT slice through the sinonasal region.
1 Pterygoid recess of the sphenoid sinus
2 Anterior clinoid process
3 Intersphenoidal septum
4 Foramen rotundum (cranial nerve V2, maxillary branch)
5 Pterygoid canal (also called the Vidian canal)

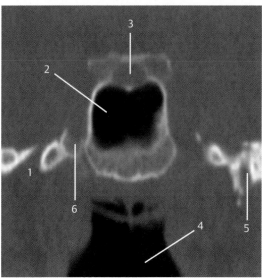

Fig. 6.12 Coronal CT slice through the sinonasal region.
1 Foramen ovale (cranial nerve V3, mandibular branch)
2 Posterior part of sphenoid sinus
3 Pituitary gland in pituitary fossa
4 Nasopharynx
5 Foramen spinosum containing the middle meningeal artery
6 Meckel cave (trigeminal ganglion of cranial nerve V)

Radiologic Anatomy on Axial CT Slices in a Craniocaudal Sequence

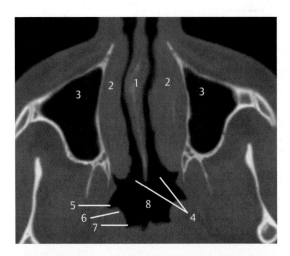

Fig. 6.13   Axial CT slice through the sinonasal region.
1 Nasal septum
2 Inferior turbinate
3 Maxillary sinus
4 Choanal opening
5 Nasopharyngeal orifice of the eustachian tube
6 Torus tubarius
7 Rosenmuller fossa
8 Nasopharyngeal space

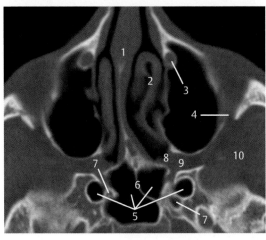

Fig. 6.14   Axial CT slice through the sinonasal region.
1 Septum
2 Curled middle turbinate
3 Nasolacrimal duct
4 Infraorbital fissure
5 Sphenoid (extended pneumatization)
6 Intersphenoidal septum
7 Internal carotid artery
8 Sphenopalatine foramen
9 Pterygopalatine fossa
10 Infratemporal fossa

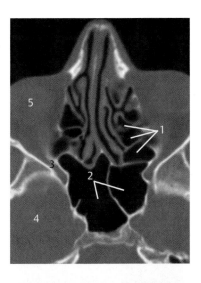

Fig. 6.15   Axial CT slice through the sinonasal region.
1 Posterior ethmoid cells
2 Sphenoid sinus
3 Infraorbital fissure
4 Middle cranial fossa
5 Ocular bulb

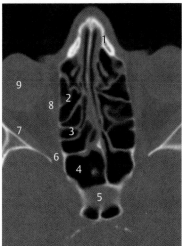

Fig. 6.16   Axial CT slice through the sinonasal region.
1 Nasal bone
2 Anterior ethmoid cells
3 Posterior ethmoid cells
4 Sphenoid sinus
5 Pituitary fossa
6 Optic canal
7 Lateral rectus muscle
8 Medial rectus muscle
9 Ocular bulb with ocular lens

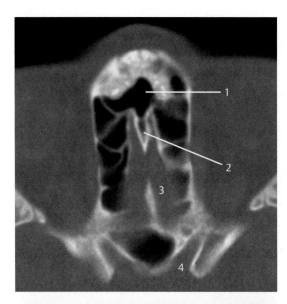

Fig. 6.17   Axial CT slice through the sinonasal region.
1 Frontal recess
2 Crista galli
3 Olfactory region (cranial nerve I)
4 Optic canal (cranial nerve II)

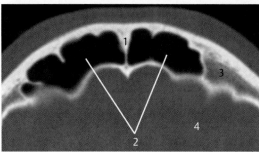

Fig. 6.18   Axial CT slice through the sinonasal region.
1 Interfrontal septum
2 Frontal sinus
3 Frontal bone containing bone marrow
4 Frontal lobe

Radiologic Anatomy on Sagittal CT Slices in a Lateral to Medial Sequence

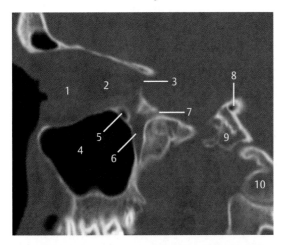

Fig. 6.19   Sagittal CT slice through the sinonasal region.
1 Ocular bulb
2 Optic nerve
3 Optic canal (cranial nerve II)
4 Maxillary sinus
5 Ethmoid cell
6 Pterygopalatine fossa
7 Foramen rotundum
8 Anterior mastoid cell
9 Sphenoid bone
10 Clivus

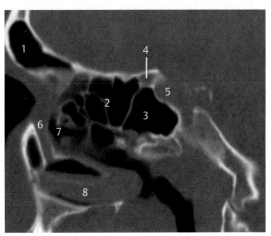

Fig. 6.20   Sagittal CT slice through the sinonasal region.
1 Frontal sinus
2 Posterior ethmoid cells
3 Sphenoid sinus
4 Optic canal
5 Pituitary fossa with pituitary gland
6 Nasolacrimal duct
7 Agger nasi cells
8 Inferior turbinate

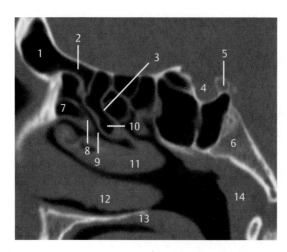

Fig. 6.21   Sagittal CT slice through the sinonasal region.
1 Frontal sinus
2 Frontal recess
3 Ground lamella (partition between the anterior and posterior ethmoid cells)
4 Pituitary fossa with pituitary gland
5 Clinoid process
6 Clivus
7 Agger nasi cell
8 Uncinate process
9 Hiatus semilunaris
10 Bulla ethmoidalis
11 Middle turbinate
12 Inferior turbinate
13 Palate
14 Adenoid

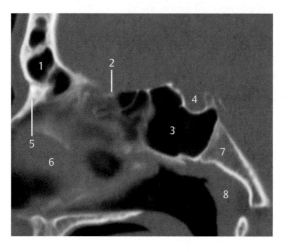

Fig. 6.22   Sagittal CT slice through the sinonasal region.
1 Frontal sinus
2 Cribriform plate and olfactory region
3 Sphenoid sinus
4 Pituitary fossa with pituitary gland
5 Nasal bone
6 Nasal septum
7 Clivus
8 Adenoid

Normal Variations of Sinonasal Anatomy

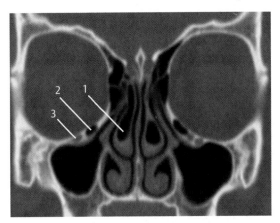

Fig. 6.23   Pneumatized middle turbinates and Haller cells.

Coronal CT slice. The middle turbinate is seen to be pneumatized on both sides (1), a normal variant that is frequently encountered unilaterally or bilaterally and is sometimes assumed to contribute to obstruction of the sinonasal outflow. Also seen on both sides is a Haller cell (2), which represents anterior extension of the ethmoid complex. In this case, the cells are situated beside the infraorbital canal (3), and confusion may arise in cases of opacification.

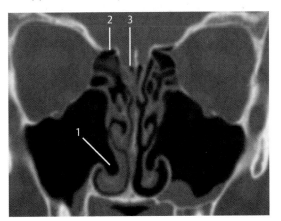

Fig. 6.24   Pneumatized inferior turbinate and low cribriform plate.

Coronal CT slice. Narrowed nasal lumen, partly due to a bilaterally pneumatized inferior turbinate (1). This rare anatomical variant presents a dilemma during surgical reduction of the turbinate, creating an inferior antrostomy in the maxillary sinus. Furthermore in this patient, note the large difference in height between the fovea ethmoidalis (2) and the cribriform plate (3), which might be a risk factor for surgical complications.

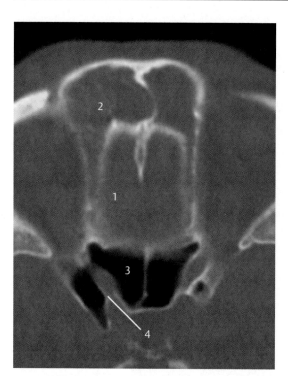

Fig. 6.25 Axial slice through the level of the olfactory bulb and optic nerve.

Axial CT slice. The olfactory bulb (1), with opacification of the frontal recess (2). In the sphenoid sinus (3), the optic nerve (4) runs freely through the sinus. This normal variant must be anticipated at surgery to prevent damage, especially in cases of opacification of the sphenoid. This risk is even higher when the nerve runs along or through an Onodi cell, which is a lateral–superior extension of the posterior ethmoid above and lateral to the sphenoid sinus. A posterior ethmoidectomy, a frequently carried out procedure, may end up with loss of vision.

7 Pathology of the Nasal Cavity and Paranasal Sinuses

Nonmalignant Pathology of the (Para)nasal Sinuses

Maxillary Sinusitis

Differential Diagnosis
- All causes of obstruction of the maxillary sinus that might induce fluid levels or persistent sinusitis.
- Periapical pathology with inflammation and osteolysis.
- Solitary (fungal) infection.
- Trauma leading to bony dislocation and obstruction of drainage from the sinus.
- Benign and malignant lesions.

Points of Evaluation
- The Waters and Caldwell views are complementary and must always be available for comprehensive evaluation and avoiding misinterpretation due to superimposition of bony structures.
- The area of the natural ostium of the sinus might be obstructed. Computed tomography (CT) can show this obstruction in more detail.
- Pay close attention to unilateral opacities, which are suggestive of tumor or odontogenic infection.
- Complete opacification may be demonstrated after previous endonasal sinus surgery, Caldwell–Luc procedures, or after orbital decompressions in Graves disease. In these patients, conventional radiography is not very useful and CT should be used for a comprehensive detailed examination.

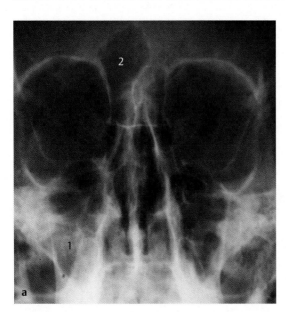

Fig. 7.1 a, b   Conventional radiographic views for sinus evaluation.

a Caldwell view. This 26-year-old patient had pain in the right maxillary region. The right maxillary sinus seems to be opacified in the lower part (1). The left frontal sinus is absent and the right frontal sinus is hypoplastic (2).

Fig. 7.1 b

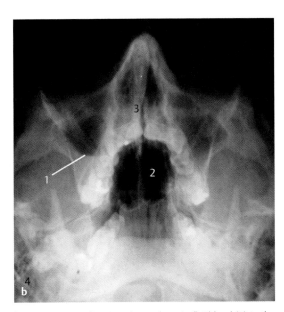

b Waters view. This view shows clear air–fluid level (1) in the right maxillary sinus seen in **Fig 7.1a**. The aeration of the maxillary sinus on the left side is confirmed. The sphenoid sinus is visible, showing normal pneumatization and aeration (2). In addition, a bony septal deviation to the right (3) is observed and there is opacification of the mastoid cells on the right side (4).

Adenoid Hypertrophy

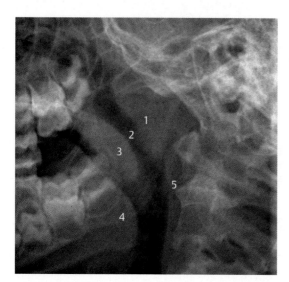

Fig. 7.2   Plain radiograph for adenoid evaluation.

Lateral skull view. Previously, in the absence of flexible endoscopes or in cases of doubt in younger children, the presence and size of the adenoid was evaluated on conventional plain films. In this lateral view of the skull, the adenoid (1) is enlarged quite extensively and almost completely obstructs the nasopharyngeal airway (2). Also seen are the velum and uvula (3), base of tongue (4), and posterior pharyngeal wall (5).

Fracture of the Nasal Bone and Retention Cysts

Differential Diagnosis
The radiologic features as seen in **Fig. 7.3** are typically pathognomic of retention cysts. In general, these retention cysts must be considered nonpathologic findings. Clinically, they are often asymptomatic or found in patients with minor complaints. In conventional radiographic views, and also on CT, these cysts may be confused with mucosal thickening of the maxillary sinus wall.

Points of Evaluation
In cases of large cysts resulting in obstruction of the maxillary sinus and those accompanied by signs of sinusitis, surgical removal (marsupialization) might be considered to improve drainage.

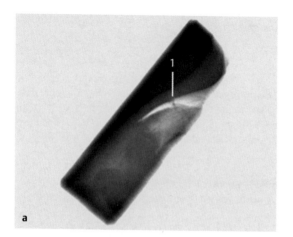

Fig. 7.3 a–c   Mild trauma to the nose. Hematoma made palpation difficult to exclude a fracture.

a Plain radiograph, lateral view. This view of the nasal bone in a patient with facial trauma demonstrates a **fracture of the nasal bone** (1), with slight depression and dislocation of the anterior part. Although the field of radiation has been restricted as much as possible, these views are not regularly taken, since palpation in most cases is sufficient to diagnose a fracture. Such radiographs may be considered in cases of severe swelling, which prevents adequate evaluation by palpation, and in cases of violence, for medicolegal reasons. CT is superior for accurate evaluation in cases of extensive facial trauma.

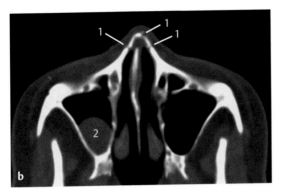

Fig. 7.3 b   Patient after facial trauma.

b CT, axial. Patient with facial trauma showing multiple fracture lines in the nasal bone (1). No other fractures were noted. A coincidence finding was a rounded lesion with smooth borders in the posterior wall of the right maxillary sinus (2). No other (mucosal) pathology of the maxillary sinus was noted. The lesion is a **retention cyst**. On coronal views (not shown), these cysts are most frequently found on the floor of the maxillary sinus.

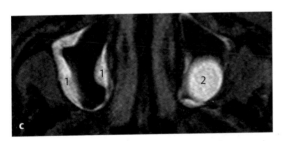

Fig. 7.3 c   Retention cysts.

c MRI, T2-weighted, axial. This patient was seen by a neurologist and complained of pressure in the region of the maxillary sinus. On the right side, the hyperintense signal (1) is indicative of mucosal thickenings adhering to the wall of the maxillary sinus. There are no signs of extensive sinusitis with no evidence of fluid levels in the sinus. On the left side, a solitary **retention cyst** (2) is seen; it is filled with hyperintense fluid and is not obviously adherent to the wall of the sinus. There is slight mucosal thickening seen in the region of the cyst.

Nasal Polyps

Differential Diagnosis

- All etiologies causing mucosal swelling and polyps.
- Chronic rhinosinusitis with or without polyps, associated with hyperreactivity, allergy, smoking.
- Less frequently: Wegener granulomatosis, which typically is associated with destruction of the nasal septum; sinonasal malignancies, which usually show infiltration of surrounding structures and/or bone destruction; and allergic fungal sinusitis.

Points of Evaluation

- Bilateral soft-tissue disease is a reassuring finding, as it usually indicates benign disease such as chronic sinusitis or polyposis.
- Anatomic structures obstructing the sinuses, due to a growth spurt in adolescence, may play a role.
- In cases with symptoms that arise later in life, concomitant secondary pathology is responsible.
- Bone destruction is the hallmark of infiltrating processes and malignant behavior.

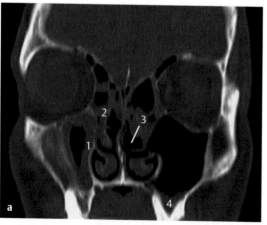

Fig. 7.4a, b   Patient with nasal obstruction, smell disorder, and rhinorrhea.

a CT, coronal. The scan shows mucosal thickening in the right maxillary sinus (1), partial opacification of the ethmoid cells (2) on both sides, pneumatization of the left middle turbinate (3), and thickened mucosa on the floor of the left maxillary sinus (4). The maxillary tooth roots are in close proximity to the floor of the sinus, which is extending down between the roots (i.e., normal finding).

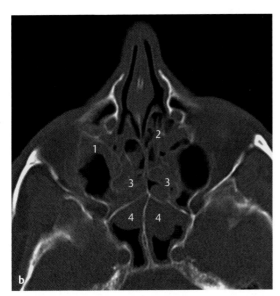

Fig. 7.4 b

b CT, axial. Mucosal thickening of the walls of maxillary sinus (1). The concha bullosa on the left side (2) is less visible on this slice. Note the opacification of the ethmoid (3) and mucosal thickening of the anterior walls of the sphenoid sinus (4) with a smooth-bordered, rounded, expansile appearance suggestive of polyps. Bone destruction is not present.

Unilateral Nasal Polyps

Differential Diagnosis

Nasal polyps, antrochoanal polyps, inverted papilloma, unilateral chronic odontogenic sinusitis with secondary polyps due to chronic infection, unilateral fungal sinusitis, mucoceles, malignancy and cystic fibrosis (similar appearance but commonly bilateral).

Points of Evaluation

- Destruction of bony outlines (with infiltrative characteristics) is suggestive of inverted papilloma, malignancies, or fungal infection.
- Calcifications in the opacified area are suggestive of fungal infection. Resorption of bone around tooth roots suggests odontogenic infection.
- Beware of pathology in the sphenoethmoidal fossa (i.e., juvenile angiofibroma).

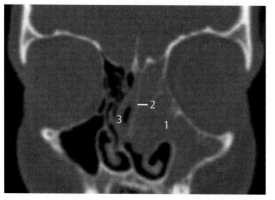

Fig. 7.5   Patient with blocked left nose.

CT, coronal. Complete opacification of the left maxillary sinus and ethmoid (1) is seen. Medial displacement of the middle turbinate (2) and nasal septum (3), indicates chronic compression of these structures. There are no signs of bony destruction of the orbital rim or the maxillary sinus or any calcifications in the opacified area.

Frontal Sinusitis

Differential Diagnosis

- Conditions causing mucosal swelling and polyps, obstructing the frontal recess.
- Unilateral processes such as inverted papilloma or malignancies.
- Fungal infections.

Points of Evaluation

- The anatomy and pathology of the frontal recess required special attention.
- In cases of persisting drainage problems in the region of the frontal recess, the septum between the frontal sinuses may be removed for establishing drainage by way of the left frontal recess.
- Bony destruction with infiltrative characteristics is suggestive of malignancy.
- Calcifications in the opacified area are suggestive of fungal infections.

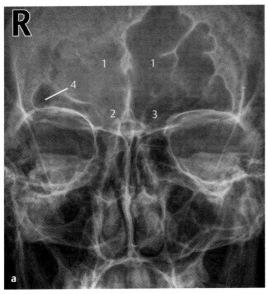

Fig. 7.6 a–c Patient with frontal headaches in the region of the right frontal sinus, with extensive pneumatization of both frontal sinuses.

a Plain radiograph, Caldwell. It is difficult to evaluate the superior aspect of the frontal sinuses (1) to determine whether these are opacified or are limited in depth. A Waters view was not helpful in discriminating depth or opacification. The frontal recess on the right side (2) seems opacified compared with the left side (3). In the most lateral part of the right frontal sinus, some aeration still seems to be present (4).

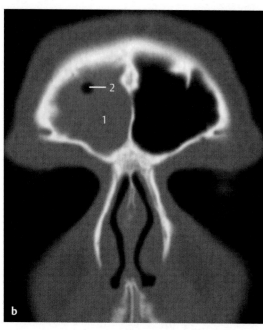

Fig. 7.6 b

b CT, coronal. Opacification of the right frontal sinus (1) is confirmed, with minimal central aeration (2). This case illustrates the point that opacification in areas of limited depth is difficult to evaluate on conventional radiography.

Fig. 7.6 c

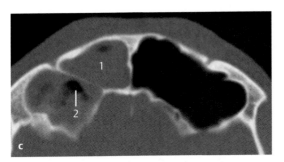

c CT, axial. Opacification (1) and partial aeration (2) of the right frontal sinus is seen. The anterior and posterior walls of the frontal sinus are intact. No calcifications are visible. An obstruction of the frontal recess may be present. In cases of failed endonasal approach, the frontal sinus and recess are easily accessible by an external approach because of sufficient length and depth of the sinus. Note: the right frontal sinus is compartmentalized by a bony septum, which may be removed for optimal drainage.

Odontogenic Sinusitis

Differential Diagnosis

Nasal polyps, inverted papilloma, unilateral chronic odontogenic sinusitis with secondary polyps, unilateral fungal sinusitis, malignancy cystic fibrosis (commonly bilateral), foreign bodies (e.g. dental filling).

Points of Evaluation

- Destruction of bony outlines with infiltrative characteristics is suggestive of inverted papilloma, malignancies, or fungal infections.
- Calcifications in the opacified area are suggestive of fungal infections.
- History of frequent dental consultations and resorption of bone around tooth roots may indicate odontogenic infections.
- Long-term antibiotics are an essential part of postoperative treatment.

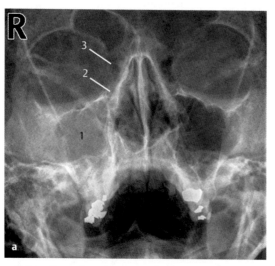

Fig. 7.7 a–c   Patient with unilateral pain and pressure in the right maxillary region.

a Plain radiograph, Waters view. There is opacification of the right maxillary sinus (1) as well as in the region of the right ethmoid (2). The right frontal recess seems slightly opacified compared with the contralateral side (3). The left side demonstrates no opacification.

Fig. 7.7 b, c

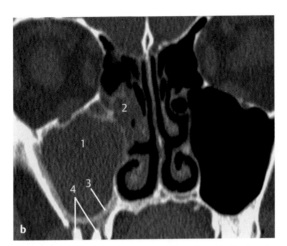

b CT, coronal. Opacification seen on CT confirms the findings in the maxillary sinus (1) and infundibulum (2). In addition, a thickened periosteal lining is observed, especially on the floor of the maxillary sinus (3). Just below this, the roots of a maxillary molar are visible (4) with signs of bone resorption, indicative of periapical infection. This is the most likely cause of the unilateral sinusitis.

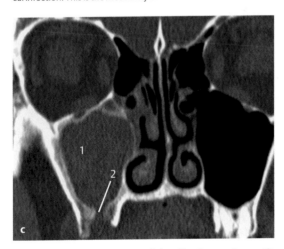

c CT, coronal. After extraction of the offending tooth, opacification of the sinus (1) and symptoms persisted due to an oroantral fistula in the maxillary bone (2). Eventually, surgical closure of this fistula cured the problem. In such cases, endoscopic sinonasal surgery may facilitate recovery.

Cystic Fibrosis

Differential Diagnosis

- All other causes of mucosal swelling and polyps, such as allergy.
- Less frequently: Wegener granulomatosis, which usually shows destruction of the nasal septum; and inverted papilloma or malignancy, often with infiltration of the surrounding bone and/or soft tissues, but rarely bilateral.

Points of Evaluation

- Destruction of bony outlines with infiltrative signs is more characteristic of malignancy.
- Expansion is more likely to be due to benign processes, such as polyposis or mucocele.
- Calcifications in the opacified area are suggestive of fungal infections.
- Resorption of bone around tooth roots indicates dental pulp infections.
- In children, expansion due to polyps can result in cosmetic problems of the exterior aspect of the nose.

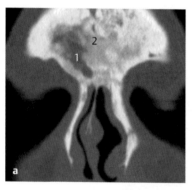

Fig. 7.8 a–c   Adult patient with known cystic fibrosis and frontal pressure feeling.

a CT, coronal. There is opacification of the right frontal sinus (1) with surrounding osteitic changes (2) such as increased thickness and sclerosis of the sinus walls. These signs are often seen in chronic infections, in particular with cystic fibrosis. In these patients, pneumatization of the frontal sinuses may be absent or limited, especially due to inflammation at an early stage during the development of the sinuses. Note the septal deviation.

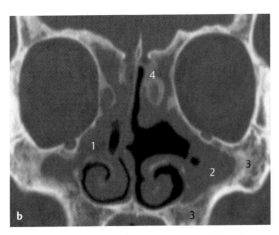

Fig. 7.8 b   Patient with cystic fibrosis history of multiple endonasal surgical procedures.

b CT, coronal. There is complete opacification of the right maxillary sinus because of re-closure of the antrostomy to the middle meatus (1), probably by polyps. The opacified left maxillary sinus (2), although a wide open antrostomy to the middle meatus is observed, is suggestive of polyps and mucosal thickening as a result of chronic inflammation. This chronic inflammation is also evidenced by the osteitic changes in the walls of the maxillary sinus (3) and ethmoid (4).

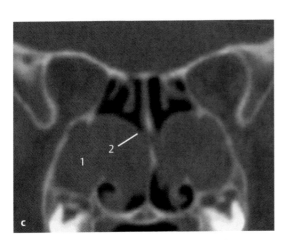

Fig. 7.8 c   CT of a 12-year-old child with cystic fibrosis.

c CT, coronal. Complete opacification of both maxillary sinuses (1), probably due to polyps and stasis of mucoid secretions. Its chronicity is demonstrated by the pressure erosion of the medial wall (2). Endoscopy of the middle meatus should reveal these polyps.

Noninvasive Fungal Sinusitis

Differential Diagnosis

All underlying causes of mucosal swelling and polyps, such as hyperreactivity, allergy, smoking. Rule out iatrogenic disorders due to extensive previous surgery. Post-traumatic lesions. Pott puffy tumor. Fistulization to the dura (cerebrospinal fluid leakage).

Points of Evaluation

- Sinusitis of the maxillary sinus, which is unresponsive to antibiotics or persists after long-term antibiotics, may be due to fungal infection. Usually, fungal infections affect the maxillary sinus. Less frequently, the frontal sinus is affected.
- Immunosuppressed patients (those with diabetes, human immunodeficiency virus [HIV] infection, or leukemia, and those taking immunosuppressive medication) are at increased risk of fungal infections.
- Opacification with general or focally increased density is suggestive of fungal infection.
- Diffuse infiltration of surrounding structures is seen in some invasive fungal infections (see also "Invasive Fungal Sinusitis," p. 240).

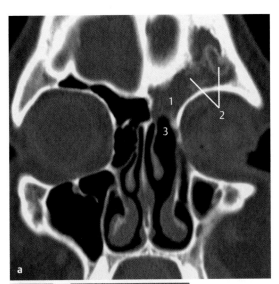

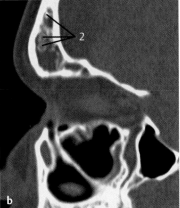

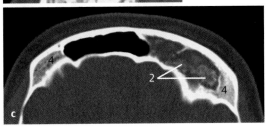

Fig. 7.9 a–c   Patient with constant left frontal sinus pressure. CT, coronal (a), sagittal (b), and axial (c). There is complete opacification of the left frontal sinus (1) in this patient, who had been previously operated on for a chronic infection (1). Within the opacified area, hyperintense, rounded or ring-shaped densities are present (2); these are most probably calcifications as are often seen in fungal infections. There are no signs of bony invasion or infiltration of surrounding structures, as is seen in more aggressive infections such as aspergillosis or mucormycosis. This patient also previously underwent drainage of the frontal recess and ethmoid (3) sinus. On both sides, more laterally in the frontal sinus on the axial slice, unaffected cancellous bone is seen (4).

Wegener Granulomatosis

Differential Diagnosis

- Other destructive causes which may, to some extent, result in destruction of the mucosa and underlying structures: chronic manipulation and crust removal by the patient, misuse of cocaine, atrophic rhinitis, sarcoidosis, and midline diseases such as lymphoma.
- Infectious diseases such as invasive fungal sinusitis, tuberculosis, and syphilis.
- Inverted papilloma and malignancies will often demonstrate a mass.

Points of Evaluation

- A history of chronic sinusitis in combination with destruction of the nasal septum is highly suggestive of Wegener granulomatosis. Pulmonary complaints and rapid improvement after steroid treatment may confirm this diagnosis. These therapeutic effects may also be observed in cases of allergic fungal sinusitis.
- Orbital involvement appears as a mass resulting in protrusion of the eyeball and diplopia (see also "Wegener Granulomatosis, Orbital Involvement," p. 247).

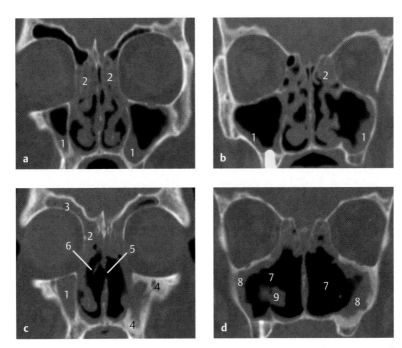

Fig. 7.10 a–d   Patient with sinus pressure, nasal discharge, crusting, hyposomia, and minor epistaxis.

a, b   CT, coronal. Some mucosal thickening is present in the maxillary sinuses (1) and ethmoid cells (2) on the anterior (left figure) and posterior slices (right figure). No signs of complete opacification or bone destruction were evident. A corticosteroid spray was given to relieve symptoms. Often, atypical changes of the mucosa can be observed in such cases.

c, d   CT, coronal. The patient's symptoms continued to worsen in the following months and a follow-up scan was taken 1 year later. CT slices, taken anteriorly and posteriorly at the same level, show a completely different picture compared with **Fig. 7.10 a, b**. The anterior slice (left figure) shows bilateral (sub)-

total opacification of the maxillary (1), ethmoid (2), and frontal (3) sinuses. There are signs of chronic infection, resulting in increased sclerosis, especially in the maxillary sinus (4). In the nasal cavity, a septal perforation (5), an osseous remnant of the right middle turbinate (6), and loss of the left middle and inferior turbinate are noted. On the posterior slice, the medial border of both the maxillary sinuses is missing (7), while the lateral border demonstrates mucosal thickening (8). Only the posterior end of the left inferior turbinate (9) is still present. Wegener granulomatosis was confirmed with laboratory tests.

Fibrous Dysplasia, Polyostotic

Differential Diagnosis

Chronic sinusitis (bacterial, fungal), cystic fibrosis, anterior skull base meningiomas, malignancies such as sarcomas, and post-radiotherapy effects.

Bone diseases: Paget disease, osteopetrosis, McCune–Albright syndrome.

Points of Evaluation

- Expansion of bone with a "ground glass" appearance and intact cortex reflects the pathophysiology of this disease (i.e., replacement of normal medullary bone by woven fibro-osseous tissue).
- A separate variant of polyostotic fibrous dysplasia is seen in McCune–Albright syndrome, with severe progressive lesions in multiple locations (also seen more often in females, and with cutaneous pigmentations and precocious puberty). See also Chapter 5, Pathology of the Skull Base.
- Secondary sinusitis and vascular or neurological deficits may develop with progression of the lesions due to encroachment of sinus ostia, fissures, skull-base foramina, and/or the optic canal. Esthetic and functional problems due to lesions in the mandible and maxilla are not uncommon.

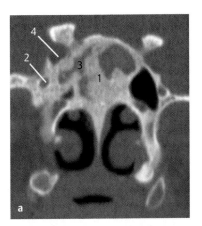

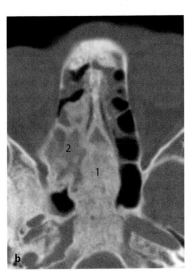

Fig. 7.11 a, b   Patient with unexplained facial pain and sinus pressure.

a CT, coronal. The sphenoid sinus is expanded and (partly) filled with hyperdense material of a so-called "ground glass" appearance (1), which is highly suggestive of fibrous dysplasia. There is compression of the foramen rotundum (2) with the possibility that the complaint of pain may be due to dysfunction of the maxillary branch of the trigeminal nerve. The remaining sphenoid sinus is completely opacified (3) due to obstruction of sinus drainage by the overgrown fibrous tissue. The right optical canal (4) (still) has a normal configuration.

b CT, axial. Note the area of the anterior skull base with extensive bone changes in the region of the olfactory bulb (1). The right posterior ethmoid area is affected as well, with central opacification of the cells (2).

Fibrous Dysplasia, Monostotic

Differential Diagnosis
Osteoma and ossifying fibroma; less likely: mucocele.

Points of Evaluation
- Expansion of bone with a "ground glass" appearance and intact cortex reflects the pathophysiology of this disease (i.e., replacement of normal medullary bone by woven fibro-osseous tissue).
- The lesion may be misinterpreted as a mucocele or an osteoma, depending on the CT window setting.
- An ossifying fibroma may demonstrate central bony densities in later stages.
- Secondary sinusitis and vascular or neurological deficits may develop with progression of the lesions due to encroachment of sinus ostia, fissures, skull-base foramina, and/or the optic canal. Esthetic and functional problems due to lesions in the mandible and maxilla are not uncommon.

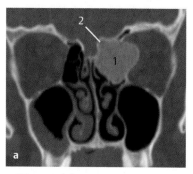

Fig. 7.12 a–c   Patient with mild proptosis and restricted ocular movements.

a CT, coronal, bone-tissue setting. A solitary lesion (1) is located in the left ethmoid and is obstructing the frontal recess with expansion into the left orbit. The left ethmoid shows expansion and has a "ground glass" appearance. The surrounding cortex is intact (2). Note the incidental mucosal thickening in the right maxillary sinus.

Fig. 7.12 b, c

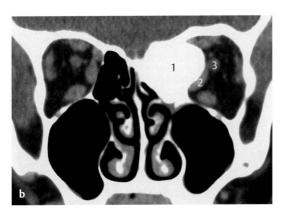

b CT, coronal, soft-tissue setting. Same patient and slice as in **Fig. 7.12 a**, different setting. There is a vast difference in the appearance of the lesion. On the soft-tissue setting (1), the lesion showed homogeneous high density, which raised the possibility of a diagnosis of osteoma or ossifying fibroma. On this setting, the intraorbital structures are better visualized with displacement of the medial rectus (2) and the optic nerve (3).

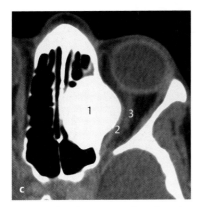

c CT, axial, soft-tissue setting. Note the mass (1) displacing the medial rectus (2) and the optic nerve (3). These appearances at different settings are suggestive for fibrous dysplasia, which was confirmed following partial surgical removal.

Osteoma

Differential Diagnosis
- Monostotic fibrous dysplasia.
- Ossifying fibroma may demonstrate central bony densities in later stages.

Points of Evaluation
Large osteomas may cause functional problems due to growth and encroachment of surrounding structures (see also section on Gardner syndrome, p. 242). For this reason, and also in small osteomas, a wait-and-scan policy might be advisable.

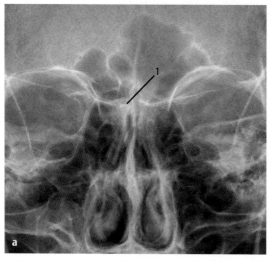

Fig. 7.13 a–c   Patient with mild headaches and frontal sinus pressure.

a Plain radiograph, Caldwell view. Stasis of secretions in the frontal recess or frontal sinus is difficult to determine on conventional radiographs, as is the small osteoma (1) that was identified on a CT scan taken later for further evaluation of pathology.

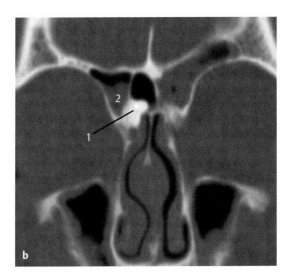

Fig. 7.13 b, c

b CT bone-tissue setting, coronal. A lesion with bone density (1) is located in the frontal recess. Behind the lesion, there is stasis of secretion (2) due to partial or complete obstruction of the frontal recess. The contralateral side also shows opacification (without signs of an osteoma). Note the mucosal thickening in the maxillary sinuses, which is probably due to an underlying cause such as allergy or hyperreactivity.

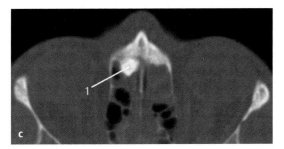

c CT, axial. Axial view through the lesion (1) located in the frontal recess. Osteomas are frequently encountered in the frontal sinus or ethmoid. Obstruction may lead to sinusitis and its complications.

Congenital Deficits

Choanal Atresia

Points of Evaluation
Most cases of choanal atresia are bony. The atresia might be incomplete or unilateral and can be associated with other congenital defects (i.e., CHARGE syndrome).

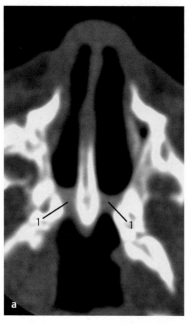

Fig. 7.14a   Neonate with respiratory distress.

a CT, axial. Both choanal areas demonstrate narrowing of the bony passage, but congenital fibrous closure (1) is the cause of the distress. Endoscopy may confirm this finding. Insufficient nasal passages in neonates results in severe dyspnea due to the obligatory nasal respiration in the first weeks, especially during feeding.

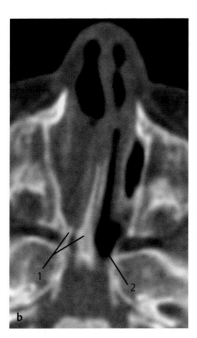

Fig. 7.14 b   Young child with complaints of right nasal obstruction.

b CT, axial. In this child, the right choanal region is completely blocked by a bony obstruction (1). Due to this deformity, the nasal septum is deviated with asymmetric growth at the level of the nasal cavity. The contralateral choanal opening has a normal appearance and opening (2) into the nasopharynx.

Piriform Aperture Malformation

Points of Evaluation

A developmental disorder of this kind may result in concomitant pathologies, such as the fusion of both maxillary central incisors to form one megaincisor (**Fig. 7.15**), in the majority of patients. Holoprosencephaly and abnormalities of the pituitary–adrenal axis are also encountered.

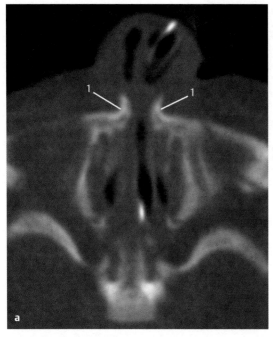

Fig. 7.15 a, b Neonate with severe dyspnea.

a CT, axial. The severe dyspnea was due to gross narrowing of the anterior nasal passage caused by bilateral bony stenosis of the piriform aperture (1).

Fig. 7.15 b

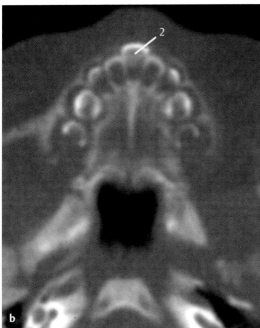

b CT, axial. Note the single central megaincisor in the upper jaw (2).

Nasolacrimal Mucocele

Differential Diagnosis and Points of Evaluation

A dilated lacrimal sac results from failure of formation of the proximal lacrimal duct; a duct mucocele results from canalization of the distal nasolacrimal duct and may appear as a soft-tissue mass under the inferior turbinate. These patients may experience recurrent inflammation of the lacrimal sac.

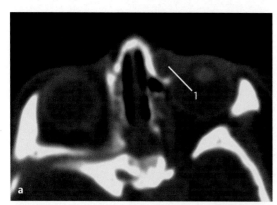

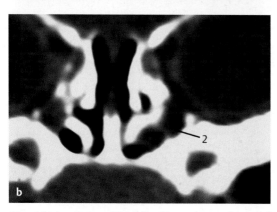

Fig. 7.16 a, b   Patient with frequent and fluctuating subcutaneous swellings below the left medial canthus.

CT, axial (a) and coronal (b). Dilated lacrimal sac in the medial canthus (1). Also, the lacrimal duct is dilated along its entire course (2), ending in the inferior meatus, probably due to distal obstruction.

Thornwaldt Cyst

Differential Diagnosis and Points of Evaluation

On MRI, the intensity varies with the protein content but is usually bright on both T1- and T2-weighted images. Usually this cyst causes no symptoms in the absence of nasopharyngeal obstruction, but patients may also present with purulent postnasal drip. These cysts rarely become infected, and if they do, they result in headaches and a stiff neck. During nasal endoscopy, a hyperemic mass of the posterior nasopharyngeal wall may be seen. Marsupialization is the definitive treatment.

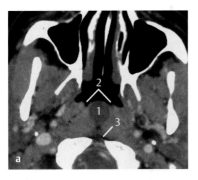

Fig. 7.17 a   Patient with hoarseness and a coincidental finding in the nasopharynx.

a CT, axial. During endoscopy, a rounded expansion on the posterior wall of the nasopharynx in a patient with sinonasal symptoms was noted. CT revealed a round, smooth-bordered cystic lesion with homogeneous nonenhancing content (1), typical of a Thornwaldt cyst. The cyst is located in the midline with the Rosenmuller fossa on both sides (2). Note the fatty pad on the prevertebral fascia (3).

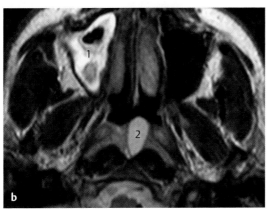

Fig. 7.17 b   This patient was referred by a neurologist for a purulent postnasal drip.

b MRI, T2-weighted, axial. A brain scan revealed hyperintense contents of the right maxillary sinus (1) due to mucosal thickening (hyperintense signal) and fluid (slightly less hyperintense). Note the hyperintense, oval, smooth-bordered cystic lesion in the posterior wall of the nasopharynx (2), also indicative of a Thornwaldt cyst.

Myxoma

Differential Diagnosis and Points of Evaluation

Fibromas present with central densities and trabeculae. Epidermoid sinus (mostly located at the tip of the nose or slightly laterally). Nasolabial cysts. Dermoid sinus (mostly in the midline), which may have a connection to the anterior fossa (enlarged foramen cecum, bifid crista galli, or broadened nasal septum), with a history of recurrent meningitis (see also "Encephaloceles," p. 174). If there is any suspicion of the latter, an MRI should be requested.

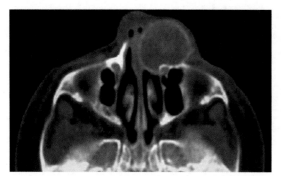

Fig. 7.18   Child, 17 months old, with a paranasal progressive swelling.

CT, axial. Bony expansion and remodeling observed on CT. Pathologic examination after complete removal revealed a myxoma.

Involvement of the Orbit

Orbital Cellulitis

Differential Diagnosis and Points of Evaluation.
See "Subperiosteal Orbital Abscess," page 239.

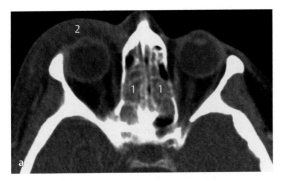

Fig. 7.19a   Patient with severe edema of the right eyelids and suspicion of orbital cellulitis.

a CT, axial with intravenous contrast. Bilateral opacification of the ethmoid (1). The lamina papyracea is intact without signs of periosteal inflammation, infiltration, or abscesses in the orbit. The only finding is preseptal edema of the right eyelid (2), which may be diagnozed as **preseptal orbital cellulitis**. The position of the eyeball is similar to the contralateral unaffected side, confirming absence of retrobulbar space-occupying pathology. Of course, facial trauma must be excluded.

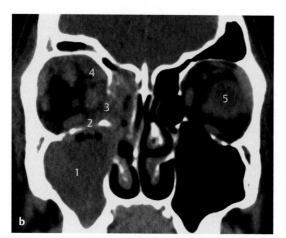

Fig. 7.19 b   Patient with a swollen red-coloured orbita on the right side and visual impairment.

b CT, coronal with intravenous contrast. On this soft-tissue setting in a patient with orbital cellulitis, who had been operated several times for sinusitis, opacification of the maxillary sinus is observed (1), with bony defects in the orbital floor (2) and lamina papyracea (3). These defects may act as a route of infection to the orbit. Along the orbital rim, enhancement can be demonstrated (4) obscuring the outer margins of the extraocular muscles. Rim enhancement (as in orbital abscess) is not seen, and there is no spread into the intraconal compartment. These signs are indicative of **diffuse orbital cellulitis**. Protrusion of the eyeball might be demonstrated on the same slice by comparing its position with that of the eyeball on the unaffected contralateral side (5).

Subperiosteal Orbital Abscess

Differential Diagnosis
Iatrogenic lesion after dacryocystorhinostomy or endonasal surgery procedures. Mucoceles. Wegener granulomatosis, invasive fungal sinusitis, Graves orbitopathy, orbital tumors or pseudotumors (nonspecific inflammatory processes), sarcoidosis. Fungal infections. Lymphoma.

Points of Evaluation
In terms of management, it is important to differentiate between preseptal cellulitis and retrobulbar disease and/or abscess (Chandler classification). As demonstrated above, imaging can be very helpful in this aspect. Rim enhancement around a central area of low density is pathognomic for an abscess. An orbital subperiosteal abscess is an emergency situation. Complications include loss of vision and cavernous sinus thrombosis.

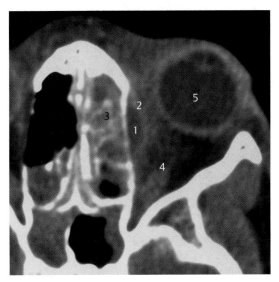

Fig. 7.20 Patient with signs of sinusitis and orbital edema.

CT, axial with intravenous contrast enhancement. The CT scan shows a **subperiosteal orbital abscess** (1) with typical rim enhancement (2). The abscess originated from infection in the left ethmoid sinus, which is completely opacified (3). Infiltrative changes in the medial orbit and around the optic nerve (4) and eyeball (5) can be noted.

Invasive Fungal Sinusitis

Differential Diagnosis
Aspergillosis, mucormycosis, inverted papilloma, odontogenic sinusitis.

Points of Evaluation
Destruction of bone with signs of infiltration is suggestive of a malignant process, especially in cases of unilateral pathology. Progressive orbital infiltration may endanger the optic nerve with loss of vision as a result. Aggressive surgical and medical eradication is mandatory.

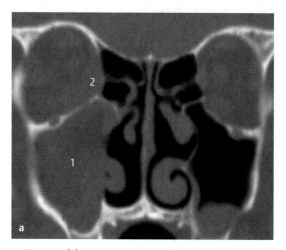

Fig. 7.21 a, b   Patient with signs of sinusitis, periorbital pain, and loss of vision on the right side.

a CT, coronal, bone-tissue setting. The bone-tissue setting reveals complete opacification of the right maxillary sinus (1), as well as very doubtful changes of the intraorbital contents along the lamina papyracea and orbital floor (2). There is no evidence of bone destruction.

Fig. 7.21 b

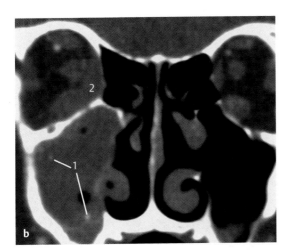

b CT, coronal, soft-tissue setting with intravenous contrast enhancement. On this setting, the contents of the maxillary sinus as well as the orbit can be evaluated much more accurately. Inside the maxillary sinus, besides the debris and mucosal thickening, small calcifications are visible (1). The orbit is infiltrated by the same pathology (2), which is suggestive of an **invasive fungal infection**. The bony outlines are not affected but may have transmitted the pathology.

Osteoma, Gardner Syndrome, and Complications

Differential Diagnosis

- May be confused with monostotic or polyostotic fibrous dysplasia.
- An ossifying fibroma may demonstrate central bony densities in later stages.

Points of Evaluation

- Extension to structures which, at surgical removal, may result in cosmetic or functional complications.
- In Gardner syndrome, multiple osteomas may be found as well as other pathologies, some of which are at an increased risk of malignancy (colorectal carcinoma and thyroid carcinoma).

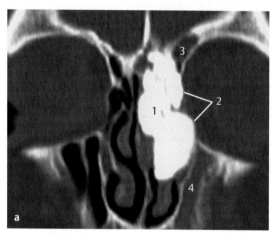

Fig. 7.22 a–c   Patient presenting with orbital cellulitis and loss of vision on the left side.

a CT, coronal, bone-tissue setting. Note the large osteoma (1) protruding through the lamina papyracea (2) and obstructing the frontal recess (3). There is opacification of the left maxillary sinus (4).

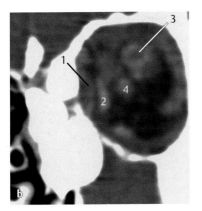
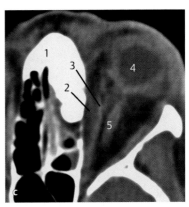

Fig. 7.22 b, c

b CT, coronal, soft-tissue setting. Enlarged view of the left orbit. There is increased density of the intraorbital fat, especially along the orbital rim, indicative of orbital cellulitis. Along the lamina papyracea, a subperiosteal abscess (1) with typical rim enhancement is present. The medial rectus (2) is displaced laterally by this abscess. A second abscess (3) is present in the intraconal compartment. The optic nerve (4) is situated near this abscess and the surrounding infiltrate, which explains the loss of vision. In this case, the osteoma was related to **Gardner syndrome**.

c CT, axial. Not the osteoma (1), subperiosteal abscess (2), and the displaced medial rectus (3). The eyeball (4) is displaced anteriorly, probably with traction on the optic nerve (5).

Mucocele

Differential Diagnosis

Polyps, meningoceles, meningoencephaloceles, esthesioneuroblastoma, or malignancies with cystic components.

Points of Evaluation

- Medical history is essential. Mucoceles are often late complications of trauma and surgery of the frontal sinus.
- Expansion and bone remodeling of an opacified sinus cavity are signs of a slow-growing lesion, and are quite typical of mucoceles. Depending on the age of the mucocele, its contents may show different signal intensities on MRI, depending on the protein content (see also Chapter 1).
- Compression of adjacent structures or the risk of bacterial invasion is an indication for total removal or marsupialization.

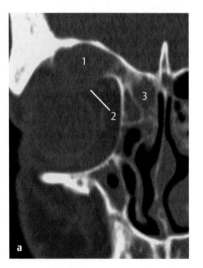

Fig. 7.23 a–e   Patient with slowly progressive proptosis of the right eye and diplopia.

a CT, coronal. The left frontal sinus is opacified with expansion of its inferior bony outline through the roof of the orbit (1). Although this is a bone-setting window, a rounded, slightly lobular, expanding lesion is seen extending from the frontal sinus toward the eyeball (2). Also, the recess and ethmoid (3) are opacified.

Fig. 7.23 b, c

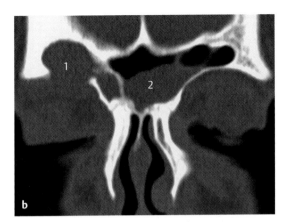

b CT, coronal. On a more anterior coronal slice, the same expansion of the frontal sinus is visible (1). In the left frontal sinus, another rounded opacity (2) is present in a partially aerated sinus.

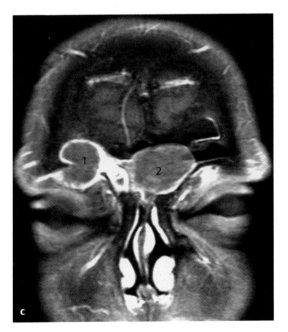

c MRI, T1-weighted with gadolinium enhancement and fat suppression, coronal. The same slice is demonstrated on MRI as previously shown on CT. Both lesions in the right (1), as well as in the left frontal sinus (2), are smooth-bordered, cystic, noninvasive lesions without contrast enhancement. The CT and MRI characteristics are suggestive of mucocele.

Fig. 7.23 d, e ▷

Fig. 7.23 d, e

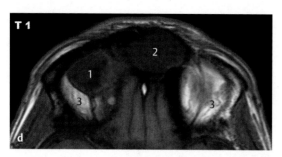

d MRI, T1-weighted, axial. The same lesions are now hypo-intense, on the right (1) with protrusion into the orbit and on the left side (2) without orbital involvement. In contrast, the periorbital fat is hyperintense (3) on this T1-weighted image.

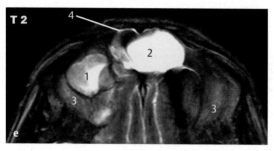

e MRI, T2-weighted, axial. On the T2-weighted image, the lesions show a hyperintense signal indicative of a high fluid content (1, 2) and confirming the diagnosis of mucoceles. The orbital fat (3) is now hypointense. The mucosal linings are hyperintense (4).

Wegener Granulomatosis, Orbital Involvement

Differential Diagnosis and Points of Evaluation
See "Amyloidosis in the Orbit," page 248.

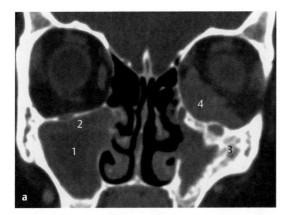

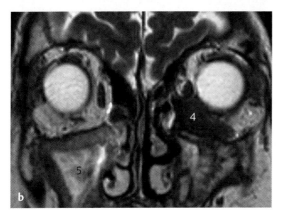

Fig. 7.24 a, b   Patient with known Wegener granulomatosis and progressive restriction of ocular movement.

CT intermediate setting (a) and MRI, T2-weighted, axial (b).
On CT, there is bilateral and complete opacification of the maxillary sinus (1), with a demarcation of the mucosal outline (2). Osseous thickening as a sign of chronic irritation is observed (3). In the left orbit, a soft-tissue mass is seen along the lamina papyracea and floor of the orbit (4). On MRI, this process has low signal intensity and seems restricted to the orbit. Biopsy revealed relapse of Wegener. In addition, the content of the right maxillary sinus is heterogeneous; centrally, the retained secretions have high signal intensity (5) while the surrounding swollen mucosa has low-to-intermediate signal intensity.

Amyloidosis in the Orbit

Differential Diagnosis

Wegener granulomatosis, invasive fungal sinusitis, orbital tumors (hemangioma, schwannoma, glioma) or pseudotumors (nonspecific inflammatory processes), myositis, localized infiltration or abscesses, sarcoidosis, infiltrated inverted papilloma.

Points of Evaluation

- Differentiation between solitary involvement of the orbit and involvement or growth from adjacent structures.
- Differentiation between unilateral and bilateral disease.
- Signs of inflammation.

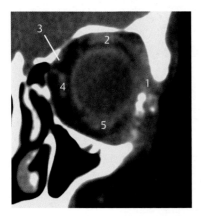

Fig. 7.25   Patient with diplopia.

CT, coronal. On this soft-tissue setting, a diffuse infiltrating lesion, also encasing and infiltrating the lateral rectus muscle, is present in the lateral orbit (1). There is destruction of the lateral orbital wall with some infiltration of the extraorbital soft tissues. Note the superior rectus (2), superior oblique (3), medial (4), and inferior (5) recti. Intraorbital biopsy revealed amyloidosis.

Anterior Skull Fractures

Points of Evaluation

- Encroachment of functional structures (ocular muscles, cranial nerves) or compression due to hematoma (orbit, subdural).
- Displacements resulting in functional (movements of the eyeball, obstruction of the nose) or cosmetic deficits.

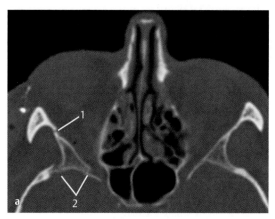

Fig. 7.26 a–c   Patient after facial trauma.

a CT, axial. The scan shows several fractures in the anterior (1) and posterior (2) right zygomatic bone due to head trauma. Clinically, proptosis may be present, due to anterior displacement of the eyeball on the affected side, as a result of orbital edema or hematoma.

Fig. 7.26 b, c

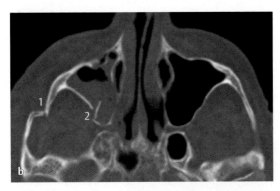

b CT, axial. On a more caudal slice from the same patient, note fractures of the zygomatic arch (1) and posterior wall of the maxillary sinus (2) with opacification of the left maxillary sinus, probably due to a hematoma.

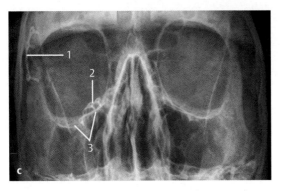

c Plain radiograph of the skull, anteroposterior view. Same patient after reconstruction of the fractures by osteosynthesis at the lateral orbital rim (1) and the orbital floor (2). There is still a step between the medial and lateral parts of the orbital floor (3).

Blow-out Fracture

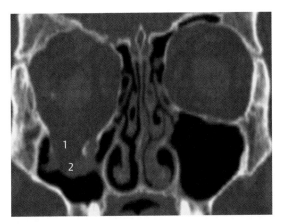

Fig. 7.27   Blunt trauma from a ball hitting the right eye.

CT, coronal. Traumatic disruption of the bony floor of the orbit (1), and prolapse of orbital fat into the maxillary sinus (2). The eyeball was at a lower level, and diplopia was noted clinically. In minor cases, small fractures might be less visible without any prolapse, but entrapment of the inferior rectus or its surrounding septated fat in these fractures might result in restriction of ocular bulb movements and diplopia.

Orbital Decompression in Graves Disease

Differential Diagnosis

Bilateral disease excludes most orbital pathology as demonstrated in previous sections, although pseudotumors are still an option.

Points of Evaluation

- Conventional sinonasal radiography in these patients is not sufficient for the evaluation of concomitant sinusitis. CT will be needed for anatomic orientation, especially if endoscopic surgery is contemplated.
- Endonasal surgical procedures must be done with care due to distortion of the normal anatomy and an increased risk of damage to displaced intraorbital structures such as the optic nerve.

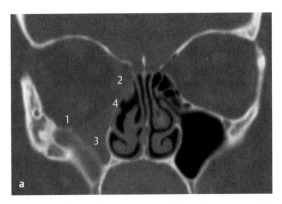

Fig. 7.28 a, b   Patient with Graves orbitopathy, after orbital decompression.

a CT, coronal. The orbital floor (1) and the lamina papyracea (2) have been completely removed. Opacification of the maxillary sinus (3) may be due to filling of orbital fat, or stasis of secretions as a result of obstruction of the drainage in the region of the natural ostium (4). In the latter case, in combination with persisting maxillary sinusitis, an antrostomy in the lower meatus may be a satisfying solution. Usually this is a standard inclusive procedure.

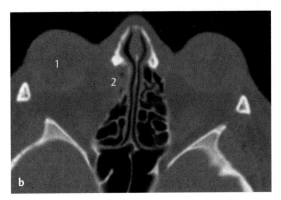

b CT, axial. Severe protrusion of the eyeball (1), despite the surgical decompression to the maxillary sinus and ethmoid (2).

Neoplasms of the (Para)nasal Sinuses

Inverted Papilloma

Differential Diagnosis
Unilateral proliferations are suspect of malignancies until the contrary is proven by biopsy. All malignant processes arising from the sinonasal cavities, nasopharynx, or the anterior skull base, and nonmalignant lesions with destructive characteristics related to compression or infiltration.

Points of Evaluation
- Accurate evaluation of involvement of intracranial structures and the surrounding vital structures such as cranial nerves or vessels (internal carotid artery, cavernous sinus) to determine treatment options and the expected morbidity.
- Radiologic differentiation and evaluation must be based on the complementary characteristics of CT and MRI.

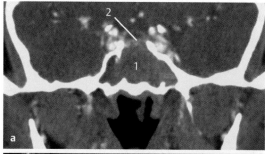
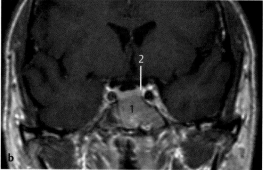

Fig. 7.29 a–d Patient operated before because of nasal polyps. Histologic evaluation revealed inverted papilloma. Follow-up scans are shown.

Fig. 7.29c

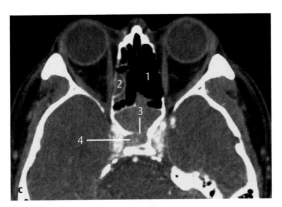

c CT with intravenous contrast, axial, soft-tissue setting. Although fine bony outlines are difficult to evaluate on this soft-tissue setting scan of the same patient as in **Fig. 7.29a**, anteriorly the left ethmoid was opened during the previous surgery and is without pathology (1). In the right posterior ethmoid, some residual pathology is likely to be present (2). The sphenoid sinus is completely opacified with osseous destruction (3) of the posterior wall and spread of disease into the pituitary fossa (4).

◁ **a, b CT with intravenous contrast (a) and MRI, T1-weighted with gadolinium enhancement (b), both coronal.** Although not considered to be truly malignant, inverted papilloma is often infiltrative and destructive in its behavior. In this patient with history of removal of an inverted papilloma, residual pathology is present in the sphenoid sinus. For accurate evaluation of the pathology (1), CT and MRI are complementary as demonstrated in these figures. On CT, destruction of the roof of the sphenoid sinus is visible (2) with possible spread to the pituitary fossa. MRI shows the outlines of the process in more detail, confirming (subtle) spread of disease (2) into the pituitary fossa.

Fig. 7.29d ▷

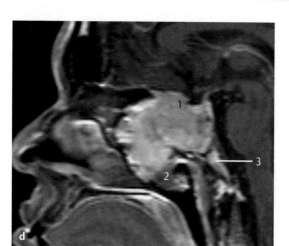

Fig. 7.29 d

d MRI, T1-weighted with gadolinium enhancement, sagittal. This sagittal view demonstrates the cranial extent of the inverted papilloma to the pituitary fossa (1), and inferior spread into the nasopharynx (2). The clivus is not (yet) infiltrated (3).

Angiofibroma, Juvenile

Differential Diagnosis

Antrochoanal polyp (peripheral enhancement only), hemangioma (usually isolated to nasal cavity, not only in adolescent males), lymphangioma, lipoma, schwannoma, neurofibroma, teratoma (present soon after birth), dermoid (fatty, cystic, polypoid), rhabdomyosarcoma (bone destruction, aggressive tumor).

Points of Evaluation

- Angiofibroma is a benign, highly vascular, nonencapsulated neoplasm that presents almost exclusively in adolescent males (aged 10–25 years). Its behavior is locally aggressive. Beside the above locations, the tumor can spread to the orbit or to intracranial structures. Also, the tumor may enhance with contrast on CT. MRI can show flow voids due to enlarged vessels within the tumor.
- Preoperative angiography and embolization to decrease blood loss during operation.
- Look for subtle deep extension because failure to identify this will lead to incomplete resection and recurrence.

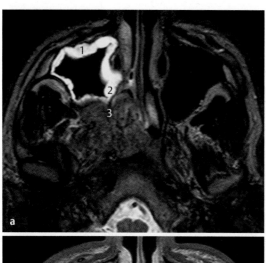
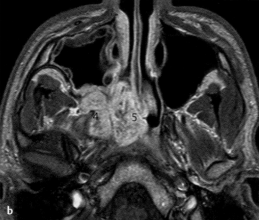

Fig. 7.30 a–d A young man with obstruction and blood-tinged nasal discharge from the right side of the nose.

a,b MRI, T2-weighted (a) and T1-weighted (b) with gadolinium enhancement. T2-weighted imaging shows hyperintense mucosal thickening (1) and probably some small retention cysts (2) in the right maxillary sinus, due to obstruction of the osteomeatal complex. Posterior to the maxillary sinus in the pterygopalatine fossa on the right side, a lesion (3) is seen bulging into the maxillary sinus (destruction of the posterior wall and part of the medial wall) and the nasopharynx, with obstruction of the choanal opening. There are no evident signs of infiltration. Post contrast administration, the lesion showed extensive enhancement due to its hypervascular nature. The location of the lesion, in the pterygopalatine fossa (4) and nasopharynx (5), and its presentation are strongly suggestive of juvenile angiofibroma. The opposite maxillary sinus shows no reactive changes because of its normal drainage.

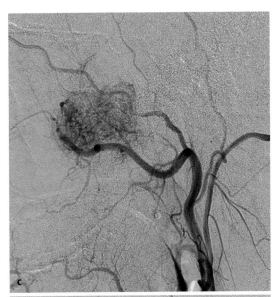

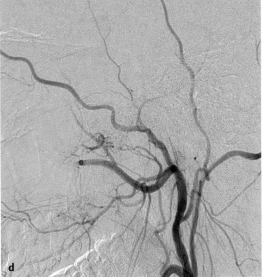

Fig. 7.30 c, d

c, d Pre- (c) and post-embolization (d) angiography. Angiography of the external carotid artery was carried out to confirm the diagnosis of juvenile angiofibroma, as well as to visualize the feeding vessels and to embolize these vessels as a preoperative procedure to facilitate surgical removal. Angiography of right external carotid artery shows an intense capillary blush of the lesion fed by the right maxillary artery. Post-embolization angiography shows marked devascularization of the lesion.

Nasopharyngeal Carcinoma

Differential Diagnosis and Points of Evaluation
See "Inverted Papilloma", page 254.

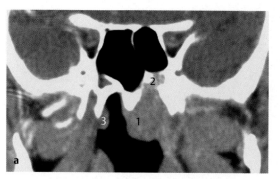

Fig. 7.31 a, b Heavy smoker with complaints of hearing loss on the left side, and mucous secretion in the middle ear at otoscopy. Nasopharyngoscopy was performed, showing a proliferation.

a CT, coronal with intravenous contrast enhancement. Note the soft-tissue mass in the roof of the nasopharynx of the left side (1), with invasion in the floor of the sphenoid (2). On the contralateral side, no disease is present. Only the torus tubarius is visible in its expected position (3). Unilateral proliferations in this area are suspicious for malignancies or lymphoproliferative pathology of the adenoid.

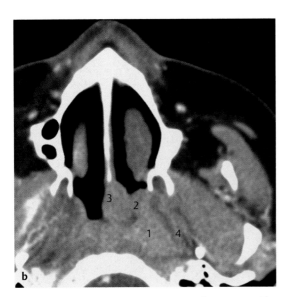

Fig. 7.31 b

b CT, axial with intravenous contrast enhancement. The same lesion (1) as seen on the previous CT, now visible on an axial view with extension to the left choanal opening (2) and posterior part of the septum (3). Obstruction of the eustachian tube (4) may resulted in unilateral fluctuating effusion into the middle ear with subsequent conductive hearing loss (at the time of scanning, no opacification of the middle ear cavity was demonstrated).

Malignancy of the Pterygopalatine and Infratemporal Fossa

Differential Diagnosis and Points of Evaluation

See "Inverted Papilloma" above. A carcinoma of the maxillary sinus may show typical perineural extension and growth into the pterygopalatine fossa and infratemporal fossa.

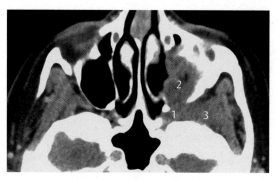

Fig. 7.32   Patient with facial pain on the left side.

CT, axial with intravenous contrast enhancement. In the pterygopalatine fossa, a lesion is seen (1) with bony destruction and invasion into the maxillary sinus (2) and the infratemporal fossa (3), suggestive of a malignancy. Note the expansion of the pterygopalatine fossa with loss of the normal fat density (when compared with the normal right side).

Neck

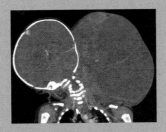

8 Radiologic Anatomy of the Neck

Computed tomography (CT) is the most commonly used imaging modality for demonstration of the neck structures. Magnetic resonance imaging (MRI) exhibits superior soft-tissue contrast. However, the quality of the MR image can be compromised by motion artifacts as a result of breathing, swallowing, and vascular pulsations.

At present, conventional radiography is still used for evaluation of swallowing disorders as well as detection of radiopaque foreign bodies. The swallowing action is discussed in a separate section at the end of this chapter.

Evaluation Points in CT of the Neck

- Asymmetry is an important point to note.
- Nasopharyngeal structures and surrounding skull base.
- Parapharyngeal space.
- Prevertebral space and fascia.
- Masticator space.
- Tongue, oral cavity.
- Salivary glands: parotid, submandibular, and sublingual glands.
- Large vessels: carotid arteries and jugular veins.
- Hypopharynx, epiglottis, vallecula, piriform sinus.
- Hypertrophic or infected lymph nodes.
- Presence of solid or cystic structures.
- Thyroid, cricoid, and true/false vocal cords.
- Trachea, esophagus, thyroid glands.
- Cervical spine.

Evaluation of the Neck Structures on Axial CT slices in a Craniocaudal Sequence

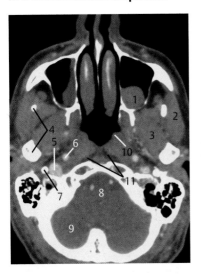

Fig. 8.1   Axial CT slice.
1 Retention cyst in left maxillary sinus
2 Masseter
3 Lateral pterygoid
4 Mandible
5 Internal jugular vein
6 Internal carotid artery
7 Styloid process
8 Pons
9 Cerebellum
10 Torus tubarius
11 Retropharyngeal space (fat)

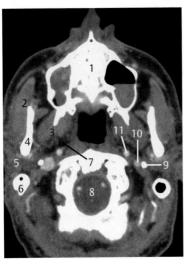

Fig. 8.2   Axial CT slice.
1 Maxilla with anterior nasal spine (*)
2 Masseter
3 Lateral pterygoid
4 Mandible
5 Parotid gland
6 Mastoid apex/process
7 Parapharyngeal space
8 Medulla
9 Styloid process
10 Internal jugular vein
     (right-sided dominance)
11 Internal carotid artery

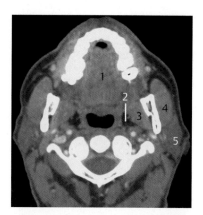

Fig. 8.3   Axial CT slice.
1 Intrinsic tongue musculature
2 Parapharyngeal space
3 Medial pterygoid
4 Masseter
5 Parotid gland

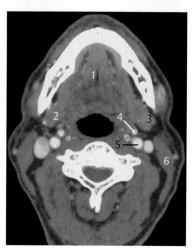

Fig. 8.4   Axial CT slice.
1 Genioglossus or geniohyoid muscle;
   may be differentiated on consecutive
   slices by their attachments
2 Submandibular gland
3 Internal jugular vein
4 External carotid artery
5 Internal carotid artery
6 Sternocleidomastoid

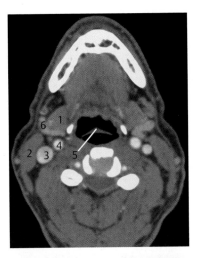

Fig. 8.5 Axial CT slice.
1 Submandibular gland
2 Sternocleidomastoid
3 Internal jugular vein
4 Common carotid artery
5 Epiglottis
6 Facial vein

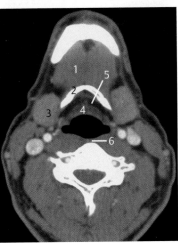

Fig. 8.6 Axial CT slice.
1 Geniohyoglossus, geniohyoid, or mylohyoid muscle; may be differentiated on
  consecutive slices by their attachments
2 Hyoid cartilage (partly ossified)
3 Submandibular gland
4 Epiglottis
5 Pre-epiglottic fat
6 Prevertebral fascia

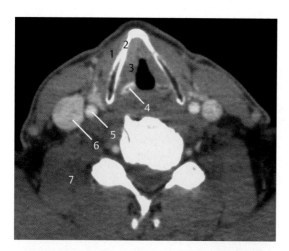

Fig. 8.7   Axial CT slice.
1 Sternothyroid
2 Thyroid cartilage
   (ossified)
3 True vocal cord
4 Arytenoid cartilage
5 Common carotid
   artery
6 Internal jugular vein
   (physiologic left/
   right asymmetry)
7 Levator scapulae

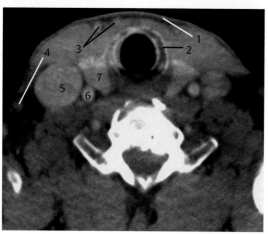

Fig. 8.8   Axial CT slice.
1 Platysma
2 Cricoid cartilage
   (partly ossified)
3 Anterior jugular vein
4 External jugular vein
5 Internal jugular vein
6 Common carotid
   artery
7 Thyroid gland
   (right thyroid lobe)

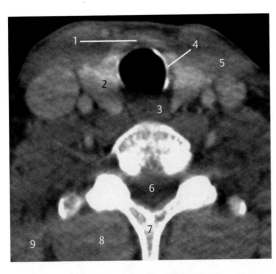

Fig. 8.9   Axial CT slice.
1. Isthmus
2. Thyroid gland (right thyroid lobe)
3. Esophagus
4. Tracheal cartilage (partly ossified)
5. Sternocleidomastoid
6. Spinal cord within the spinal canal
7. Vertebra (spinous process)
8. Semispinalis cervicis
9. Levator scapulae

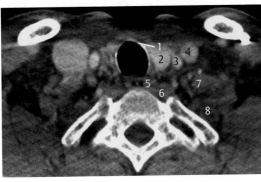

Fig. 8.10   Axial CT slice.
1. Tracheal cartilage (partly ossified)
2. Thyroid gland (left thyroid lobe)
3. Common carotid artery
4. Internal jugular vein
5. Esophagus
6. Longus colli
7. Scalenus anterior
8. Scalenus medius and scalenus posterior

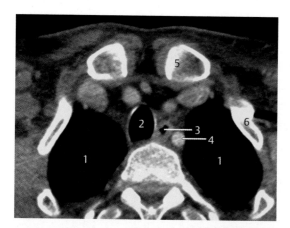

Fig. 8.11   Axial CT slice.
1 Apex of lung
2 Tracheal lumen
3 Esophageal lumen
4 Left subclavian artery
5 Clavicle
6 First rib

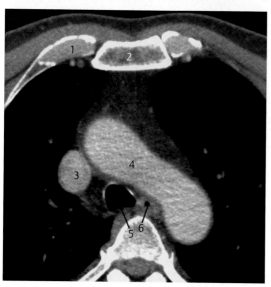

Fig. 8.12   Axial CT slice.
1 First rib
2 Sternum
3 Superior vena cava
4 Aortic arch
5 Trachea
6 Esophagus

Evaluation of the Neck Structures on Coronal CT Slices in an Anteroposterior Sequence

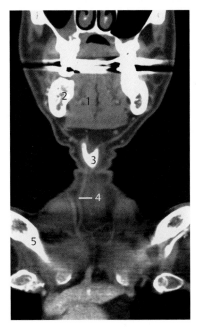

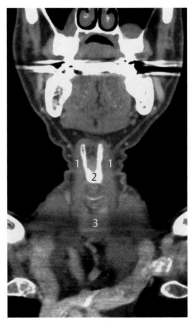

Fig. 8.13   Coronal CT slice through the neck.
1 Genioglossus or geniohyoid muscle; may be differentiated on consecutive slices by their attachments
2 Mandible
3 Hyoid cartilage (partly ossified)
4 Anterior jugular vein
5 Clavicle

Fig. 8.14   Coronal CT slice through the neck.
1 Prelaryngeal ("strap") muscles
2 Hyoid cartilage (partly ossified)
3 Isthmus of thyroid gland

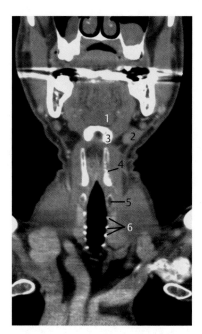

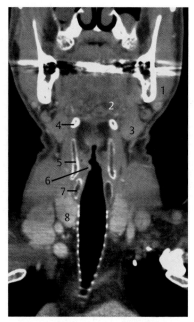

Fig. 8.15   Coronal CT slice through the neck.
1 Genioglossus
2 Submandibular gland
3 Hyoid cartilage (partly ossified)
4 Thyroid cartilage (partly ossified)
5 Cricoid cartilage (partly ossified)
6 Tracheal cartilage rings (partly ossified)

Fig. 8.16   Coronal CT slice through the neck.
1 Parotid gland
2 Sublingual gland
3 Submandibular gland
4 Hyoid cartilage (partly ossified)
5 Thyroid cartilage (partly ossified)
6 True vocal cord
7 Cricoid cartilage (partly ossified)
8 Thyroid gland (right thyroid lobe)

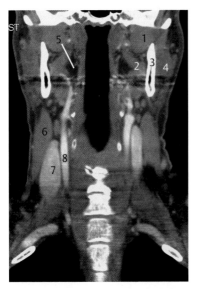

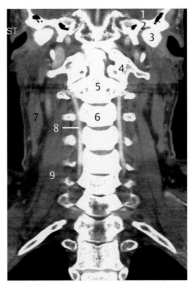

Fig. 8.17 Coronal CT slice through the neck.

1 Lateral pterygoid
2 Medial pterygoid
3 Mandible
4 Masseter
5 Parapharyngeal space
6 Sternocleidomastoid
7 Internal jugular vein
8 Common carotid artery

Fig. 8.18 Coronal CT slice through the neck.

1 Middle cranial fossa
2 Petrous bone
3 Mandibular condyle
4 Atlas
5 Axis
6 Cervical spine (C3)
7 Sternocleidomastoid
8 Vertebral artery
9 Scalene musculature (deep musculature)

Conventional Radiography of Swallowing Problems

For evaluation of swallowing problems, a video recording of the entire radiologic examination to evaluate the dynamics of deglutition is the best option.

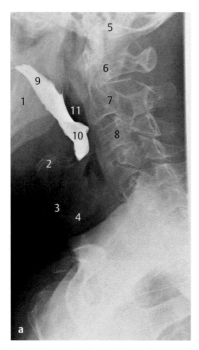
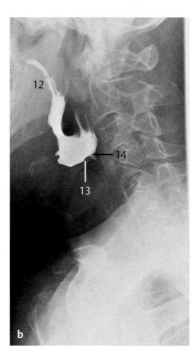

Fig. 8.19 a–g   Radiographic evaluation of swallowing problems.

a–d Lateral series. For anatomic orientation, we have indicated the mandible (1), hyoid (2), thyroid (3), cricoid (4), occipital bone (5), atlas (6), axis (7), and the third cervical vertebra (8).

The contrast passes from the oropharynx (9) to the hypopharynx (10), by the action of the stripping wave as a result of contraction of the hypopharyngeal musculature (11). A moment later, the contrast is pushed out of the oropharynx by the base of the tongue (12), with stasis above the epiglottis (13) which is not yet fully closed (14).

Then the distal part of the hypopharynx opens (15) and, with relaxation of the cricopharyngeus muscle and the upper esophageal sphincter (16), the contrast passes into the esophagus (17). There are no signs of aspiration in the subglottic region (18) or in the posterior part of the trachea (19).

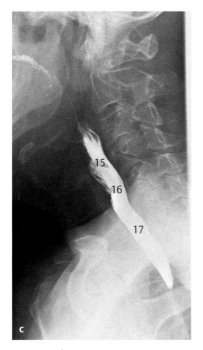
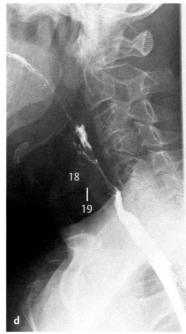

Fig. 8.19 c, d

Fig. 8.19e–g ▷

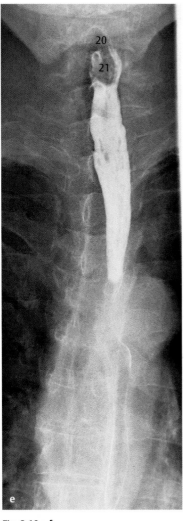 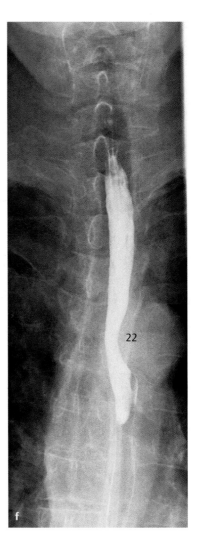

Fig. 8.19 e, f

e–g Anteroposterior series. On this series, the more distal stages of contrast passage can be observed. Although not visible in this patient, after passage from the hypopharynx (20), occasionally there is stasis of contrast in the vallecula in the area of the thyroid (21). On a lower level, the physiologic narrowing of the esophagus due to pressure from the aortic arch (22) compresses the contrast column before it enters the distal esophagus (23).

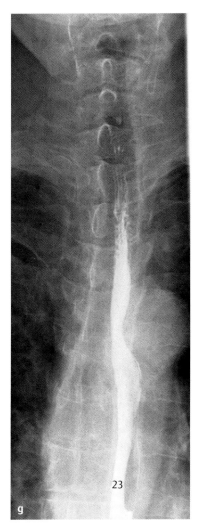

Fig. 8.19 g

9 Pathology of the Neck

Pathology of the Suprahyoid Neck

Tonsillar Abscess

Differential Diagnosis
- Severe and acute Epstein–Barr infection.
- In unilateral cases: spread of infection from an odontogenic or parapharyngeal abscess.
- More likely without clinical signs of infection: asymmetric lymphoid hyperplasia, tonsillar retention cyst (fluid collection without capsular enhancement), lymphoma (e.g., non-Hodgkin), malignancies.

Points of Evaluation
- Lymphoproliferative growth of other lymph nodes in cases of systemic infection or lymphoma, infiltrative signs.
- Beware of airway obstruction and spread to parapharyngeal spaces, cavernous sinus (thrombosis), or cervical (pre)vertebral areas.

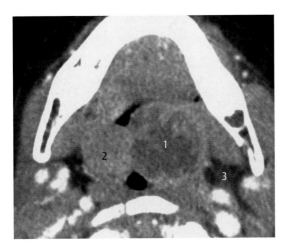

Fig. 9.1   This 4-year old child had severe bilateral tonsillitis with symptoms of a left peritonsillar abscess.

CT with intravenous contrast enhancement, axial. The left tonsil (1) is much larger than the contralateral side (2) with central hypodensities suggestive of necrosis or fluid collections, confirming the presence of an abscess. The abscess is still limited to the tonsil, that is, there are no signs of peritonsillar spread. However, the parapharyngeal fat on the left side shows mildly increased density (3), indicative of edema and/or cellulitis. In this case, the tonsils were removed immediately because of airway obstruction.

Tonsillar Carcinoma

Differential Diagnosis
Chronic infections with unilateral lymphadenitis (human immunodeficiency virus [HIV], syphilis, tuberculous tonsillitis, Plaut–Vincent), granulomatous diseases, aphthous diseases, parapharyngeal abscess, lymphoma.

Points of Evaluation
- Staging is based on enlarged or pathologic-appearing lymph nodes, bilaterality, and spread of tumor to the contralateral side.
- Because of the involvement of lymph nodes, infections might also be considered. However, the unilateral presentation excludes systemic infections.
- Lymphomas initially might present as unilateral lymphadenopathy.

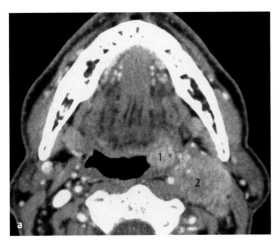

Fig. 9.2 a, b Patient with complaint of pain in the oral cavity and left neck region.

a CT with intravenous contrast enhancement, axial. In the left tonsillar fossa, a small and enhancing tumor is visible (1), with enlarged level II lymph nodes (2) highly suggestive of metastasis. The internal jugular vein is not visible, probably due to the enlarged lymph nodes.

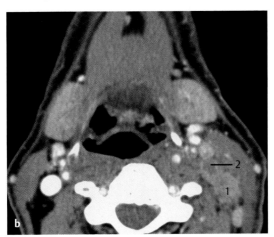

b CT with intravenous contrast enhancement, axial. Same patient as in **Fig. 9.2 a**, slice at a lower level, of the epiglottis. This area (i.e., level III) also shows enlarged lymph nodes (1), some with central necrosis (2).

Oropharyngeal Tumor, Base of Tongue

Differential Diagnosis
Benign and malignant tumors (squamous cell, salivary glands), lymphoma, granulomatous diseases (Wegener, sarcoidosis), infections (HIV, syphilis, tuberculous, Plaut–Vincent).

Points of Evaluation
- Staging by enlarged or pathological-appearing lymph nodes, bilaterality and spread of tumor to the contralateral side.
- Lymphomas (non-Hodgkin) initially may present as unilateral lymphadenopathy and ulcerative lesions.
- Evaluation of systemic disease and lymph nodes in other regions as well as secondary tumors in the hypopharynx and larynx.
- Keep in mind that (micro)metastases may be radiographically occult.

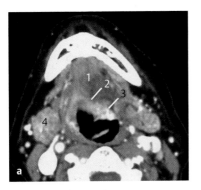 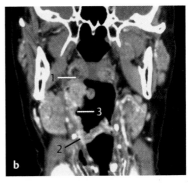

Fig. 9.3 a–c   Patient with globus sensation and some referred pain to the right ear.

a CT with intravenous contrast enhancement, axial. Axial slice at the level of the mandible and floor of the mouth (1). At clinical evaluation, an ulcer was found at the base of the tongue on the right side. The depth of this lesion (2) is quite well visualized on CT, with enhancement of the margins extending to the contralateral side (3) and the ipsilateral posterior side (4). This was staged as a T3N2c oropharyngeal tumor (enlarged lymph nodes not depicted).

b CT with intravenous contrast enhancement, coronal. The upper border (1) of the lesion, at the level of the soft palate, as well as the lower border (2) in the vallecula are clearly visualized, together with the ulcer at the center of the tumor (3).

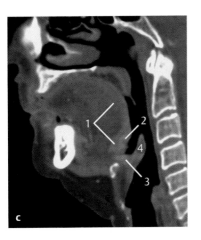

c CT with intravenous contrast enhancement, sagittal. The sagittal view of the tongue shows the extent and depth of the lesion at the base of the tongue (1), its ulcerative surface (2), and infiltration into the vallecula (3). Whether the epiglottis (4) is affected remains unclear from this image. No infiltration of the pre-epiglottic space is present.

Multiple Synchronous Malignancies

Differential Diagnosis
Malignancies (squamous cell, salivary glands), diseases of the Waldeyer ring: lymphoma, granulomatous diseases (Wegener, sarcoidosis), infections (HIV, syphilis, tuberculous, Plaut–Vincent)

Points of Evaluation
- Staging is based on enlarged or pathologic-appearing lymph nodes, bilaterality, and spread of each tumor to the contralateral side.
- Lymphomas (non-Hodgkin) initially may present as unilateral lymphadenopathy and ulcerative lesions.
- Evaluation of systemic disease and lymph nodes in other regions.
- Keep in mind that (micro)metastases may be radiographically occult.

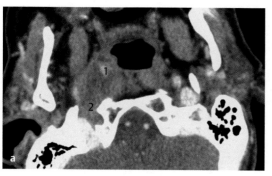

Fig. 9.4 a–c Heavy smoker and alcohol abuse with complaints of a sore throat.

a CT with intravenous contrast enhancement, axial. A lesion with malignant characteristics is seen in the right tonsillar fossa (1). The internal jugular vein on the right side, often dominating the view, might be occluded by direct invasion or thrombosis (2). The carotid artery is compressed.

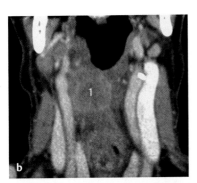

Fig. 9.4 b, c

b CT with intravenous contrast enhancement, coronal. In the same patient, another tumor is also noted in the hypopharynx (1). Both the common carotid artery and internal jugular vein are patent at this level.

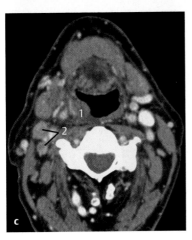

c CT with intravenous contrast enhancement, axial. The axial view through the hypopharyngeal lesion (1) shows multiple ipsilateral lymph nodes are enlarged, some of them with central necrosis (2), indicative of metastasis.

Abscess of the Neck

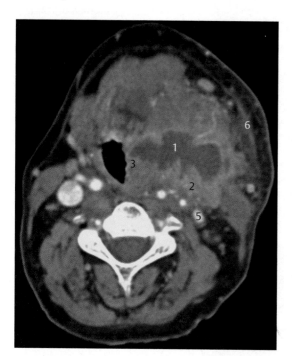

CT with intravenous contrast enhancement, axial. A large abscess (1) with a thick, contrast-enhanced capsule (2). The abscess is extending to the hypopharyngeal wall (3), with compression of the hypopharyngeal lumen, resulting in a severe inspiratory stridor. This slice is taken at the level of the base of the tongue (4). The left internal jugular vein (5) is much smaller than on the right side, probably due to partial compression by the abscess or physiologic asymmetry. The infiltration of the subcutaneous fat and thickened platysma on the left side (6) are suggestive of infection or edema.

Parapharyngeal Abscess

Differential Diagnosis
Necrotizing lymph node metastases, lymphadenitis, mycobacterial infections, infected (epi)dermoid cyst or branchial cleft cyst, laryngocele (usually lower level).

Points of Evaluation
- The radiographic sign indicating involvement of the parapharyngeal spaces is the disappearance or compression of fat.
- Beside the important clinical features of infection, the hypodense contents of the lesion and its contrast-enhancing wall help in making the diagnosis of an abscess.
- Beware of the danger of airway obstruction and spread to the parapharyngeal spaces, the cavernous sinus (thrombosis), or the cervical (pre)vertebral areas.

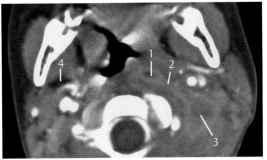

Fig. 9.6 Patient with fever, trismus, and pain on swallowing.

CT with intravenous contrast enhancement, axial. Note the bulging left pharyngeal wall, as a result of a parapharyngeal abscess (1) which is spreading (2) to deeper structures in the neck (3). In contrast to the contralateral side, the fat in the parapharyngeal space is not visible on the affected side (4). A different window setting may better illustrate the enhancing wall of the abscess.

Lymphadenitis Colli

Differential Diagnosis

Reactive lymphadenopathy. Various primary infective agents: bacterial, viral, fungal, mycobacterial, toxoplasmosis, cat-scratch disease, syphilis. Neoplastic lymphoma. Sarcoidosis (sometimes with calcifications). Metastases with central necrosis.

Points of Evaluation

- Infected lymph nodes usually show homogeneous enhancement.
- Cavitation may indicate mycobacterial infections or necrotizing metastases.
- Beware of spread of infection outside the lymph nodes (parapharyngeal spaces, cavernous sinus thrombosis).

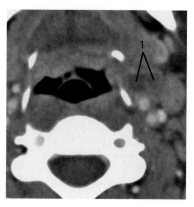

Fig. 9.7   Patient with pyrexia of unknown origin and signs of infection in the neck.

CT with intravenous contrast enhancement, axial. Various enlarged level III lymph nodes are present near the internal carotid artery and jugular vein. Some of them show central necrosis (1), with slight rim enhancement. Although blood tests were indicative of bacterial infection no causative microorganism was isolated, and the patient was successfully treated with broad-spectrum antibiotics.

Lymphadenopathy, HIV

Differential Diagnosis
See Lymphadenitis.

Points of Evaluation
HIV infections may be associated with coexisting lymphoma and chronic lymphadenitis. Coexisting diseases may have a different clinical presentation in HIV.

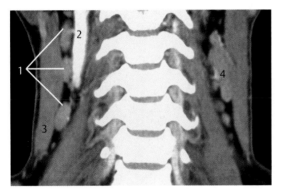

Fig. 9.8 Young male patient with episodes of fever and sweating during the night and enlarged cervical lymph nodes of unknown cause.

CT with intravenous contrast enhancement, coronal. Serology revealed HIV infection. On the right side, multiple homogeneously enhancing enlarged lymph nodes (1) are seen along the carotid artery and jugular vein (2), medial to the sternocleidomastoid muscle (3). On the left side, besides multiple solitary nodes, an enhancing conglomerate of lymph nodes (4) is observed.

Lymphoma, Non-Hodgkin

Differential Diagnosis
- Other neoplastic lymphomas: Hodgkin disease, chronic lymphatic leukemia.
- For non-neoplastic causes, see "Lymphadenitis Colli", page 288.

Points of Evaluation
Look for non-Hodgkin disease in extralymphatic sites such as the nasopharynx and tonsils. Hodgkin disease tends to be localized. On CT and MRI, non-Hodgkin disease usually presents as enlarged lymph nodes with homogeneous contrast enhancement. Central necrosis is typically associated with a higher likelihood of malignancy.

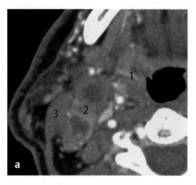 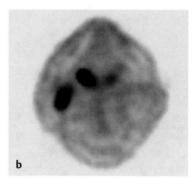

Fig. 9.9 a–d   Patient with enlargement and ulceration of the right tonsil as well as cervical lymph node enlargement.

a CT with intravenous contrast enhancement, axial. On this slice, an area of different structure with enhancement is seen at the base of the tonsillar fossa (1). A conglomerate of deep cervical lymph nodes (2) demonstrating non-homogeneous enhancement and central hypodensities are seen at level II, medial to the sternocleidomastoid muscle (3).

b PET, axial. The positron emission tomography (PET) scan shows enhanced uptake at both locations as seen on the CT. No further hot spots are present. A biopsy confirmed non-Hodgkin B-cell lymphoma of the right tonsil.

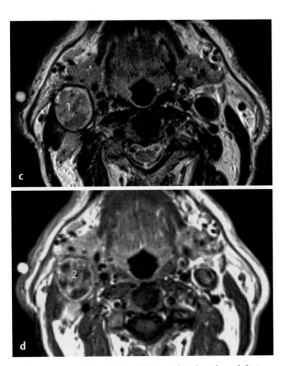

Fig. 9.9 c, d

c, d MRI, T2-weighted (c) and T1-weighted with gadolinium enhancement (d), axial. At a lower level, the level II lymph node has a nonhomogeneous appearance on the T2-weighted image (1), which is confirmed by heterogeneous uptake of contrast (2). The capsule of the lymph node is intact (i.e., there are no signs of extracapsular spread). Histopathologic evaluation revealed a non-Hodgkin lesion.

Carotid Body Paraganglioma

Differential Diagnosis

Glomus vagale, jugulotympanic paraganglioma, hemangiopericytoma, salivary gland tumors, schwannoma, or neurofibroma (very rare). Less likely due to their hypodense nonenhancing contents: branchial cleft cysts, lymphangioma, dermoid cysts, lipoma.

Points of Evaluation

- Glomus vagale may be accompanied by displacement of the internal and external carotid arteries, however, it is not localized to the carotid bifurcation but rather to the parapharyngeal spaces in most cases. Dysfunction of cranial nerves IX, X, and XI may be associated with this pathology, especially in cases of jugulotympanic paraganglioma, which primarily occurs in the region of the jugular foramen and also can be associated with tinnitus.
- Tumor may be present in multiple locations in (familial) paraganglioma as well as in neurofibromatosis.

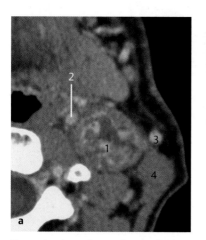 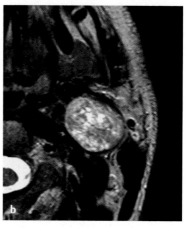

Fig. 9.10 a–d   Patient with a slowly progressive lesion in the neck.

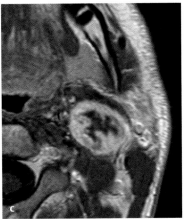

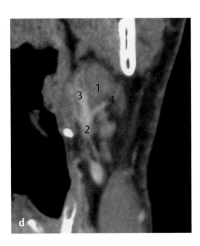

Fig. 9.10 c, d

a–c CT with intravenous contrast enhancement, axial (a), MRI, T2-weighted, axial (b), and T1-weighted, axial (c). Slices through the left side of the neck at the level of the lower border of the mandible. A smooth-bordered, rounded lesion (1) with a heterogeneous appearance (salt-and-pepper) is visible. On T2-weighted images the tumor displays mixed signal intensities. The enhancing parts have signal intensities equivalent to muscle, while the more cystic, nonenhancing areas demonstrate high signal intensities. There is strong heterogeneous enhancement both on CT and on MRI. The tumor is situated between the internal and external carotid arteries, a characteristic location. The internal jugular vein is not visible, probably due to compression. Also seen are the internal carotid artery (2), facial vessel (3), and the sternocleidomastoid (4).

d CT with intravenous contrast enhancement, coronal. The coronal view shows the lesion (1) located at the bifurcation of the common carotid artery (2). Note also the internal (3) and external (4) carotid arteries. This is a classic picture of a carotid body paraganglioma.

Branchial Cleft Cyst

Differential Diagnosis

Laryngocele, cystic hygroma (septations), lymphoma or metastases with central necrosis (frequently multiple nodes), and dermoid cyst (fat content). Diagnoses less likely due to the appearance of the lesion in **Fig. 9.11** are abscess (surrounding infiltration), hemangioma or paraganglioma, and lipoma.

Points of Evaluation

- If present, the internal opening of the cleft cyst is situated in the tonsillar fossa (second branchial cleft) or in the superior part of the piriform sinus (third branchial cleft).
- Other possible differential diagnoses may need to be considered depending on the presence of septal structures inside the lesion, presence of a thickened and irregular capsule with signs of surrounding infiltration, and the density of the content.
- Papillary thyroid carcinoma has a propensity for cystic-appearing lymph node metastases. When single, such a node may present as a branchial cleft cyst.

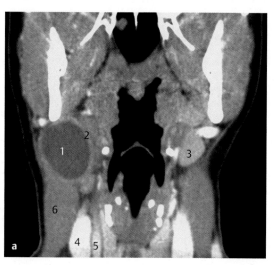

Fig. 9.11 a, b   Patient with a periodically fluctuating swelling of the right neck without further complaints.

CT with intravenous contrast enhancement, coronal (a) and axial (b).

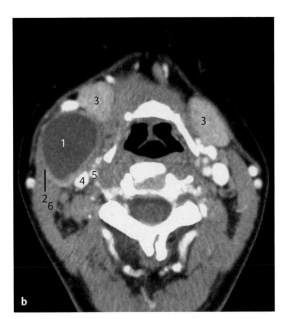

Fig. 9.11 b

Note the hypodense, cystic, smooth-bordered structure (1) with an enhancing capsule (2) that is thickened, probably due to lymphocytic infiltration or infections in the past. This location is typical for a branchial cleft cyst. In general, it is situated behind the submandibular gland (3), lateral to the jugular vein (4) and external carotid artery (5), and in front of the sternocleidomastoid (6), where the fistula, if present, frequently opens.

Cystic Hygroma, Lymphangioma

Differential Diagnosis

- In mild cases the lesion might be discovered as an incidental finding on radiology. In these cases other diagnoses are possible: branchial cleft cyst, laryngocele, salivary gland disorders (sialadenitis).

  Less likely and depending on the appearance of the lesion and its content are: small abscesses, necrotizing lymph node metastases, lymphadenitis, neoplastic lymphoma, mycobacterial infections, hemangioma, paraganglioma, schwannoma, dermoid cyst, lipoma

Points of Evaluation

- Signs of previous infections, compression of vital structures and risk of airway obstruction, vascular compromise or neurologic deficits.
- In neonates, lymphangioma might grow rapidly and extensively, resulting in considerable deformities.

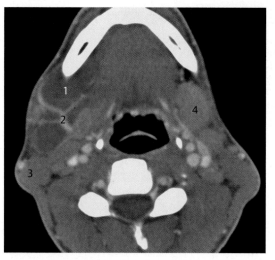

Fig. 9.12   Patient with stable swellings of the neck, without any medical complaints but with some aesthetic deformity.

CT with intravenous contrast enhancement, axial. There is hypodense multilobular cystic structure (1) at the level of the mandible with medial displacement of the submandibular gland. Internal enhancing septations (2) are present in the lesion, which has no clear surrounding capsule. In this case, the sternocleidomastoid (3) is situated posterior to the lesion. Contralateral submandibular gland (4)

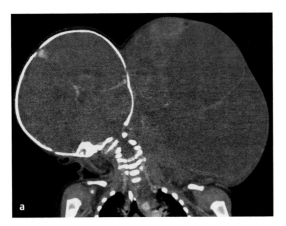

Fig. 9.13 a, b Neonate with an extensive cystic hygroma of the head and neck.

a CT with intravenous contrast enhancement, coronal. During the first weeks, the lesion enlarged rapidly and, due to compression of the trachea, a tracheostomy was necessary.

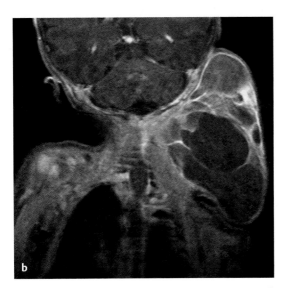

b MRI, T1-weighted with gadolinium enhancement, coronal. Note the heterogeneous contents of the lesion in the left neck and its enhancing septations. The largest part of the lesion is not enhanced due to the predominant fluid content. Ultrasound can be useful for initial evaluation of such lesions.

Pathology of the Infrahyoid Region of the Neck

Supraglottic and Pharyngeal Tumors

Differential Diagnosis
Benign and malignant tumors (squamous cell, salivary glands), papillomatosis, lymphoma, granulomatous diseases (Wegener, sarcoidosis), infections (HIV, syphilis, tuberculous).

Points of Evaluation
- Staging is based on enlarged or pathologic-appearing lymph nodes, bilaterality, and overgrowth of the tumor on the contralateral side.
- Lymphomas (non-Hodgkin) initially might present as unilateral lymphadenopathy and ulcerative lesions.
- Evaluation of systemic disease and lymph nodes in other regions as well as secondary tumors in hypopharynx and larynx.
- Keep in mind that micrometastases may be radiologically occult.

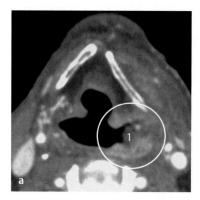 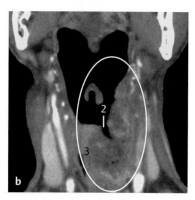

Fig. 9.14 a, b   Patient with pain in the throat and coughing after swallowing.

a CT with intravenous contrast enhancement, axial. Axial slice at the level of the thyroid cartilage shows a soft-tissue mass (outlined as indicated) centered in the left piriform sinus with nonhomogeneous enhancement and irregular mucosal surface (1).

b CT with intravenous contrast enhancement, coronal. The coronal slice demonstrates the extent of the lesion (outlined as indicated) with an ulcerative crater (2), deep caudal growth and extension over the midline to the right side (3), all suggestive of a large **piriform sinus carcinoma**. The tip of the epiglottis serves as an anatomic landmark that can be used in endoscopic biopsies to confirm the diagnosis.

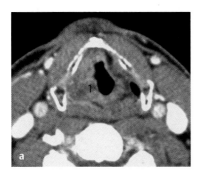
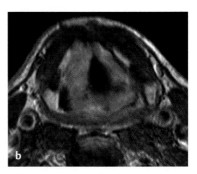

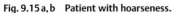

Fig. 9.15 a, b   Patient with hoarseness.

a, b CT with intravenous contrast enhancement (a) and MRI, T1-weighted with gadolinium enhancement (b), both axial. Slices at the level of the false vocal cords show an asymmetric appearance of the endolaryngeal tissues, due to a right **false vocal cord tumor** (1). In this case, MRI demonstrates no additional informa-tion. Note: absence of paralaryngeal fat on the right side is indicative of deep infiltration. There is irregular ossification of the thyroid cartilage on both sides and no signs of cartilage destruction and/or extralaryngeal spread. This is (somewhat) better appreciated on the MR image due to superior soft-tissue contrast.

Supraglottic Tumor

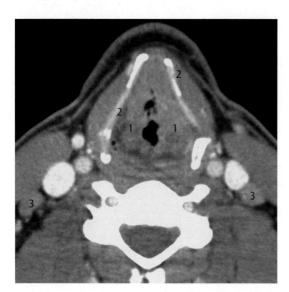

CT with intravenous contrast enhancement, axial. The lesion extends bilaterally (1), highly indicative of a malignancy. The nonhomogeneous appearance of the thyroid (2) may be a normal finding indicative of partial ossification of the thyroid cartilage, or may be a sign of invasion of the thyroid, indicating a malignancy. Bilaterally behind the jugular vein, homogeneous, slightly enlarged lymph nodes (3) are seen.

Glottic Tumor

Differential Diagnosis
Chronic laryngitis due to several causes, papillomatosis, Wegener granulomatosis.

Points of Evaluation
- Staging is based on enlarged or pathologic-appearing lymph nodes, bilaterality, and overgrowth of the tumor on the contralateral side.
- Destruction, infiltration, and unilateral pathology are considered a malignancy until a diagnostic biopsy provides evidence to the contrary.

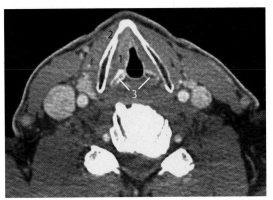

Fig. 9.17 Patient with hoarseness.

CT with intravenous contrast enhancement, axial. Slight asymmetry of the vocal cords can be observed with slight enlargement of the vocal cord on the right side including the anterior commissure (1). The right thyroid lamina shows a small area of erosion (2) of the inner cortex (i.e., T3 stage). Small portions of the arytenoids are also visible (3). The right arytenoid shows (mild) sclerosis compared with the normal left side.

Thyroglossal Duct Cyst

Differential Diagnosis
Congenital cervical dermoid, goitrous thyroid, (para)thyroid nodules or tumors, lymphadenopathy, salivary gland cysts, external laryngocele (protrusion through the thyrohyoid membrane), cystic metastases.

Points of Evaluation
- The thyroglossal duct runs from the tongue to the region of the thyroid, and cystic remnants most frequently occur below or at the level of the hyoid. A thyroglossal duct cyst might be located in the midline or slightly off the midline and has a characteristic relation to the strap muscles.
- Presence of a normal and functional thyroid gland should be confirmed before removal of the cyst. Look for signs of invasion in case of suspected malignancies. Ultrasound usually provides sufficient information by establishing the cystic nature of the lesion and the presence of a normal thyroid gland.

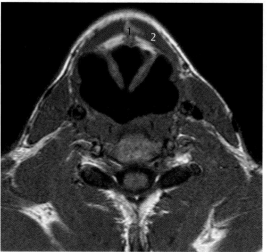

Fig. 9.18   Patient with a fluctuating swelling in the anterior part of the throat.

MRI, T1-weighted, axial. Small lesion (1) with high signal intensity on T1-weighted images, probably due to presence of protein-rich fluid, situated in the midline at the level of the hyoid. The lesion is embedded in the prelaryngeal strap muscles (2). All features are suggestive of a small thyroglossal duct remnant.

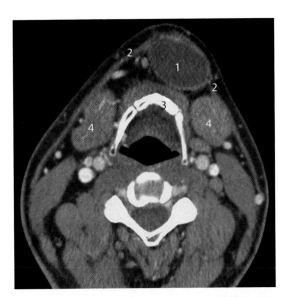

Fig. 9.19 Asymptomatic slowly progressive swelling anterior to the throat.

CT with intravenous contrast enhancement, axial. Cystic lesion (1), slightly off midline in close relation to the prelaryngeal strap muscles (2), in front of the hyoid (3), and at the level of the submandibular glands (4). The cyst is filled with low-density fluid, characteristic of a thyroglossal duct cyst. Previous infections or hemorrhage may result in a thick enhancing rim.

Hypertrophy of the Thyroid Gland, Thyroid Goiter

Differential Diagnosis

Lesions that are not uniformly distributed on both sides: thyroid gland nodules and malignancies (most frequently papillary carcinoma), lymphoma, metastases. Solitary lesions may represent a thyroglossal duct cyst or a congenital cervical dermoid.

Points of Evaluation

- CT and MRI are useful to determine retrosternal extension and tracheal compression.
- Malignancies might show invasion of the surrounding structures, lymphadenopathy, and metastases but could also be intrathyroid, which can be misinterpreted as thyroid nodules.
- Calcifications, as often seen in thyroid cancer, are rare in thyroid lymphoma.
- Beware of metastases from other structures to the thyroid.

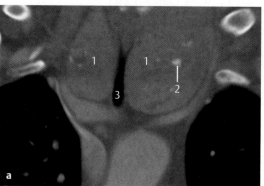

Fig. 9.20 a–c   Slowly progressive bilateral swelling with some feelings of dyspnea.

a CT with intravenous contrast enhancement, coronal. This slice at the level of the lower neck/upper thoracic cavity, shows enlarged thyroid lobes (1) with the nonhomogeneous appearance and coarse calcifications (2) typical of thyroid goiter. Progressive enlargement may compress the tracheal lumen (3) and result in stridor and respiratory difficulties.

Fig. 9.20 b, c

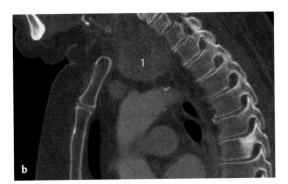

b CT with intravenous contrast enhancement, sagittal. The goiter is located dorsally and partly retrosternally (1) and is associated with a higher risk of tracheal and/or esophageal compression compared with goiter that is located more anteriorly and cranially in the neck.

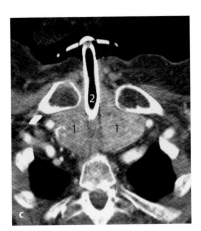

c CT with intravenous contrast enhancement, axial. Intermediate-to-strong contrast enhancement with a slight nonhomogeneous appearance of both enlarged thyroid lobes (1), due to high vascularity. In this case, compression of the trachea warranted a tracheostomy and placement of a cannula (2). The cannula is enclosed by the goiter.

Note: Bone-setting window was used for **Fig. 9.20 a** and **b**, but a soft-tissue setting would have allowed better evaluation.

Laryngeal Trauma

Points of Evaluation

In acute trauma, endolaryngeal edema and/or hematoma may cause progressive airway obstruction. Sometimes, a temporary tracheostomy is necessary. Such emergencies are among the few situations in which a noncontrast-enhanced CT of the neck is indicated.

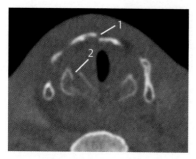

Fig. 9.21   Young male patient with blunt trauma to the larynx resulting in a hoarse voice and pain.

CT, axial bone window. CT at the level of the glottis showed multiple fractures; this figure shows a midline fracture with slight inward displacement of the partly ossified thyroid cartilage (1). There is a second fracture, with minor dislocation, of the right lamina of the cricoid cartilage (2). These fractures, in combination with post-traumatic edema, entrapment of air and/or hematoma, are the cause of the voice disorder. The dislocations were repositioned surgically.

Pathology of the Salivary Glands

Sialadenitis

Differential Diagnosis
Acute sialadenitis due to bacterial or viral infections, as well as chronic sialadenitis. These might be secondary to dehydration, immunosuppression, obstruction by sialoliths, post-radiotherapy, Sjögren syndrome or sarcoidosis, granulomatous diseases.

Points of Evaluation
- Sialography, now mostly considered to be an obsolete procedure, is not always informative but may show irregular duct ectasia, expansion, or stenosis. It is contraindicated in acute sialadenitis as it may exacerbate inflammation.
- In Sjögren syndrome, a nonhomogeneous pattern on CT is seen due to interstitial fibrotic changes and calcifications.
- In sarcoidosis there is lymphadenopathy and pulmonary/mediastinal involvement.

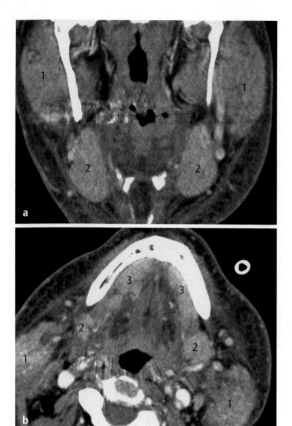

Fig. 9.22 a, b Patient with chronic intermittent enlargement of the salivary glands and diffuse pain.

CT with intravenous contrast enhancement, coronal (a) and axial (b). There is diffuse enlargement of all salivary glands: the parotid glands (1), submandibular glands (2), and the sublingual glands (3). Local areas of low density suggestive of abscess formation or stasis of secretions are not visible. No hyperdensities suggestive of calcifications or concrements are present.

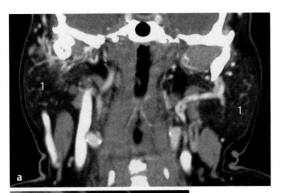

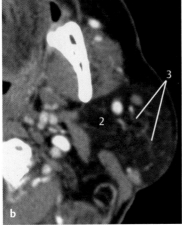

Fig. 9.23 a, b   Young male patient with acute bilateral parotitis due to mumps. CT with intravenous contrast enhancement, coronal (a) and axial (b). The coronal CT shown extensive swelling of both parotid glands (1). An enlarged axial view of the left side shows marked hypodensity of the parotid parenchyma (2) and increased intraglandular vascularity (3). These findings may be because of the acute infection and hyperemia. Again, no abscess formation or sialoliths are present.

Sialolith of the Submandibular Gland

Differential Diagnosis
See "Sialadenitis," page 307.

Points of Evaluation
Be aware that sialoliths may also be radiolucent; bimanual palpation is an adjunctive diagnostic tool.

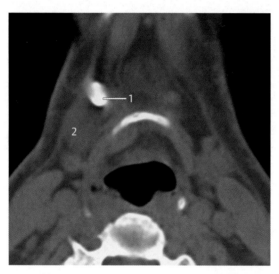

Fig. 9.24   Patient with fluctuating complaints of swelling and pressure feeling in the right submandibular region.

CT, axial bone window. A hyperdensity (1), with similar density as bone, suggestive of a sialolith (stone, calculus), probably obstructin outflow of the duct. The submandibular gland is also seen (2).

Pleomorphic Adenoma of the Submandibular Gland

Differential Diagnosis

Cystadenolymphoma (Warthin; heterogeneous due to protein-rich or hemorrhagic cysts), lipoma, schwannoma, lymphangioma. Malignancies may be easily overlooked using radiologic evaluation alone.

Points of Evaluation

- Calcifications are well depicted on CT, as are signs of infection and abscess formation. On CT, most pleomorphic adenomas are smooth-bordered, spherical, benign-looking tumors that usually display a higher density than the surrounding parotid parenchyma. Sometimes, these tumors demonstrate a heterogeneous appearance with sites of lower attenuation representing areas of necrosis, old hemorrhage, and/or cystic change (see **Fig. 9.25**).
- For MRI characteristics, see "Pleomorphic Adenoma of the Parotid Gland," page 316.

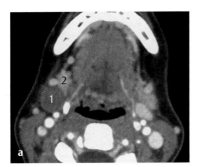 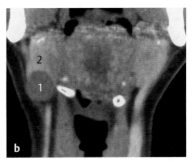

Fig. 9.25 a, b Patient with an asymptomatic slowly progressive swelling in the right submandibular region. Shaving his beard off revealed this pathology.

CT with intravenous contrast enhancement, axial (a) and coronal (b). There is a well-delineated mass with homogeneously hypodense content (1) in the posteroinferior part of the right submandibular gland (2).

Ranula of the Sublingual Gland

Differential Diagnosis
- Branchial cleft cysts, cystic hygroma, thyroglossal duct cyst.
- Less likely due to the contents: (epi)dermoid cysts, lipoma.
- May be misinterpreted as a widened submandibular duct due to obstruction (sialolith) or infection (sialodochitis).

Points of Evaluation
The content provides an important differentiating radiologic sign, as are the course and location of the lesions mentioned above. Occasionally a ranula will extend into the parapharyngeal space.

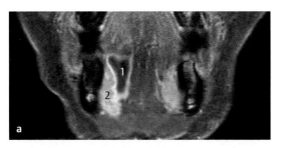

a MRI, T1-weighted with gadolinium enhancement and fat suppression, coronal. There is a cystic lesion suggestive of a ranula (1), originating from the superior part of the right sublingual gland (2). A ranula is not a true cyst (lined by epithelium) but a fluid collection in connective tissue.

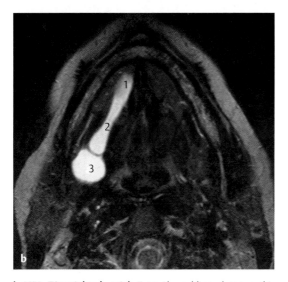

b MRI, T2-weighted, axial. From the sublingual space, this plunging ranula (1) extends through the mylohyoid muscle with a characteristic small connection (2), the so-called tail-sign, to a larger portion (3) situated in the submandibular space.

Lipoma Near the Parotid Gland

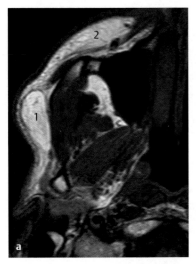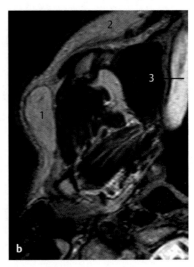

Fig. 9.27 a, b   Asymptomatic weak swelling in the parotid region.

a, b MRI T1-weighted (a) and T2-weighted (b), axial. The smooth-bordered, ovoid lesion in and near the parotid gland area (1), with its thin, surrounding capsule and high intensity signal on T1- and T2-weighted imaging, is suggestive of fat. Compare it with the subcutaneous fat (2), which also has high signal on T1- and T2-weighted imaging. The T1- and T2-weighted images can be differentiated by the hyperintense appearance of the inferior turbinate (3). The lesion did not enhance with gadolinium (not shown). All findings are suggestive of a benign lipoma of the neck. Fine needle aspiration was used to confirm this diagnosis.

Cholesteatoma Near the Parotid Gland

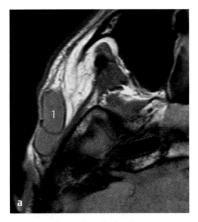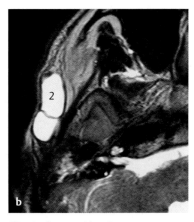

Fig. 9.28 a, b   Soft and slowly progressive swelling in the parotid region.

a, b MRI, T1-weighted (a) and T2-weight-ed (b), axial. There is multilobulated, smooth-bordered lesion superficially within or near the parotid gland. The homogeneous content is isointense with brain tissue on the T1-weighted image without contrast (1). On the T2-weighted image, however, the lesion is hyperintense similar to cerebrospinal fluid, indicating fluid-rich contents (2). Surgery was undertaken based on suspicion of a parotid tumor, which revealed keratin contents suggestive of cholesteatoma.

The patient's history included two surgical procedures on the right middle ear for removal of cholesteatoma. A slight indication for this can be seen on the T2-weighted image with some hyperintense content of the mastoid. Re-evaluation of the MRI after surgery revealed a **cholesteatoma** extending from the middle ear through the subcutaneous tissue to the parotid region. In this case, fine needle aspiration would have been helpful in making a preoperative diagnosis.

Pleomorphic Adenoma of the Parotid Gland

Differential Diagnosis
- Cystadenolymphoma (Warthin; heterogeneous on T1- and T2-weighted images due to protein-rich or hemorrhagic cysts), lipoma (hyperintense on T1-weighted images, hyperintense on T2-weighted images), schwannoma, lymphangioma.
- For malignancies of the parotid gland, see next section.

Points of Evaluation
Pleomorphic adenoma represents approximately 75% of all parotid tumors. They have a slow growth pattern and occasionally present with a characteristic lobulated appearance. They may become aggressive and malignant. A high rate of recurrence after surgery might be ascribed to microscopic extensions.

For the evaluation of a suspected parotid pleomorphic adenoma, gadolinium enhancement does not provide more information, but, if used, it must be done with fat suppression because of the high content of fat within the parotid gland.

For CT characteristics, see "Pleomorphic Adenoma of the Submandibular Gland", page 311.

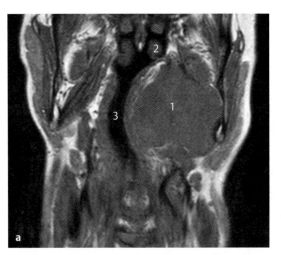

Fig. 9.29 a–c   Slowly progressive swelling of the neck and swallowing problems.

a MRI, T1-weighted, coronal. Note the extensive, isointense, smooth-bordered lesion (1) in the hypopharyngeal area: from the level of the floor of the nasal cavity (turbinates, 2) protruding into and partially obstructing the airway (3) at the level of the oropharynx.

Fig. 9.29 b, c

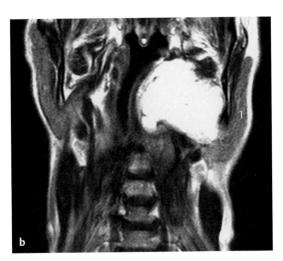

b MRI, T2-weighted, coronal. The lesion is hyperintense on a T2-weighted image, with no signs of invasion into the surrounding structures. The lesion could have originated from the deep part of the parotid gland or the parapharyngeal accessory salivary glands. The superficial parotid lobe seems intact (1). The lesion is protruding extensively into the oropharyngeal lumen, but it is not extending towards the exterior cheek.

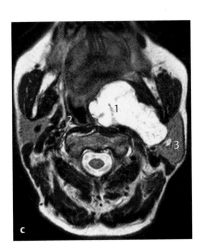

c MRI, T2-weighted, axial. The lesion is occupying the parapharyngeal space (1), as compared with the normal contralateral side (2). The major part of the parotid seems intact (3). These figures suggest a pleomorphic adenoma, the most frequent salivary gland tumor, mostly originating from the parotid gland. This was confirmed at pathological evaluation after surgical excision.

Malignancies of the Parotid Gland

Differential Diagnosis

Mucoepidermoid carcinoma, adenoid cystic carcinoma, acinic cell carcinoma, and malignant mixed tumors are the most frequently occurring malignant epithelial tumors. As well as these tumors, nonepithelial tumors (sarcoma, lymphoma) and metastases (squamous cell, renal cell, thyroid) must be kept in mind.

Points of Evaluation

- MRI is superior to CT in the evaluation of parotid gland tumors, although it has low specificity for differentiation between tumors. Gadolinium enhancement may help in evaluation of perineural growths. If used, fat suppression is necessary because of the high fat content within the parotid gland. Solid processes (low signal on T1- and T2-weighted images) are more suggestive of malignancy. The degree of sharpness of the outline does not help differentiate between benign and malignant lesions unless significant invasion in surrounding structures is noted.
- CT better defines calcifications as well as signs of infection. Ultrasound, with or without fine needle aspiration, is usually sufficient to assess superficial small tumors. For deeper and larger tumors, MRI is recommended.
- From a surgical point of view, the facial nerve is situated between the superficial and deep lobe of the parotid gland. Superficial tumors are associated with less risk of facial nerve damage at surgical removal.
- Low-grade mucoepidermoid carcinoma might show cystic lesions, but the higher grades of malignancy are more solid and difficult to differentiate from pleomorphic adenoma. Keep in mind that although a pleomorphic adenoma can behave in a benign way for years, it may become malignant with aggressive infiltration and metastases (i.e., carcinoma from a pleomorphic adenoma); tumors in nonparotid sites (such as palate, paranasal sinuses) have higher rates of malignancy.

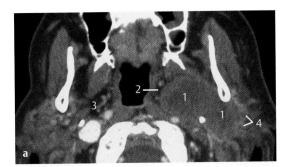

Fig. 9.30 a, b Slight swelling of the left parotid region and deep pain.

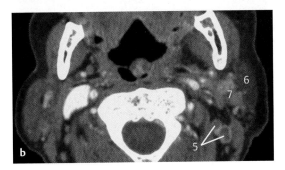

CT with intravenous contrast enhancement, axial. On the left, a large solid lesion (1) is extending from the deep parotid lobe. Laterally, this process is not sharply outlined. The parapharyngeal fat is displaced (2) compared with the contralateral side (3). The tumor appears to be quite homogeneous, although some cystic structures may be present (4). At a lower level, lymph node metastases with central necrosis and capsular enhancement are seen (5). Furthermore, the parotid tail (6) is partly infiltrated by the tumor (7). This appearance is suggestive of a **malignant mixed tumor,** such as **mucoepidermoid** or **adenoid cystic carcinoma**.

Adenoid Cystic Carcinoma

Differential Diagnosis and Points of Evaluation
See previous section.

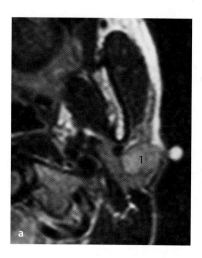
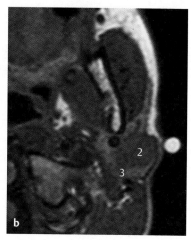

Fig. 9.31 a–c   Patient with a painless swelling of the left parotid region. MRI evaluation was requested. Before the MR study, the location of the lesion was marked on the skin. These images of the parotid region illustrate the different characteristics of MR images and the use of gadolinium enhancement. With fat suppression, the normal glandular signal drops due to the high fat content of parotid parenchyma, allowing differentiation from the enhancing tumor. After surgical removal, this tumor was revealed to be an **adenoid cystic carcinoma**, a tumor also found in other salivary glands. Its prognosis strongly depends on its histologic pattern, perineural growth, bone invasion, and presence of distant metastases.

a MRI, T2-weighted. Limited lesion within the boundaries of the parotid gland. The T2-weighted image (1) demonstrates a uniform high-to-intermediate signal intensity.

b MRI, T1-weighted. T1-weighted imaging without gadolinium enhancement demonstrates the characteristic low intensity of the lesion (2) compared with the surrounding normal parotid tissue (3).

Fig. 9.31 c

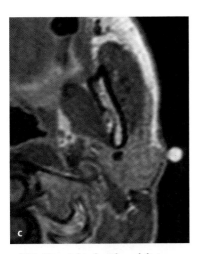

c MRI, T1-weighted with gadolinium enhancement. On T1-weighted imaging with gadolinium enhancement, the tumor seems to have disappeared due to equal enhancement of the normal parotid parenchyma and the lesion. Therefore, if gadolinium enhancement is required for evaluation of an intraparotid lesion, it is recommended to also use fat suppression.

Acinic Cell Carcinoma

Differential Diagnosis and Points of Evaluation
See previous section.

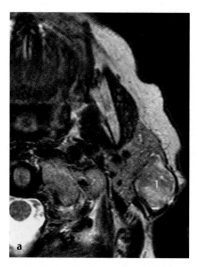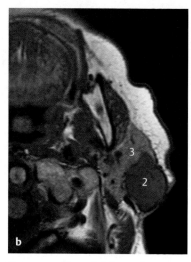

Fig. 9.32 a–c Another patient with a parotid tumor with well-delineated contours located in the posteroinferior part of the gland.

a MRI, T2-weighted without gadolinium enhancement, coronal. Heterogeneous signal intensity (1) without evident cystic structures.

b MRI, T1-weighted without gadolinium enhancement, coronal. Low intensity without gadolinium enhancement (2) compared with the surrounding normal parotid tissue (3).

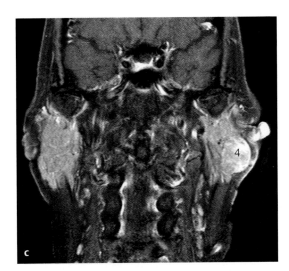

Fig. 9.32 c

c MRI, T1-weighted with gadolinium enhancement and fat suppression, coronal. Strong enhancement after administration of gadolinium (4). After surgical removal, this tumor was revealed to be an **acinic cell carcinoma** with low-grade malignant potential. This tumor is predominantly found in the parotid gland.

Pathology of the Esophagus and Thoracic Cavity

Aspiration

Differential Diagnosis
In other cases, swallowing problems may be because of: strictures caused by chemically induced trauma or surgical interventions, foreign bodies, hypertrophy of the cricopharyngeal muscle, Zenker diverticulum, laryngocele, compressive or infiltrative tumors from the esophagus or surrounding structures.

Points of Evaluation
- Occasionally aspiration is caused by mechanical failure of the epiglottis to close because of the presence of tumor, but most cases are due to neurologic (sensory) disorders without any visible pathology apart from the aspiration. Beware of aspiration pneumonia.
- The above-mentioned pathologies are partly demonstrated in other sections.

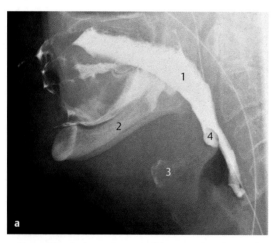

Fig. 9.33 a–c Swallowing problems are best evaluated radiographically by fluoroscopy with simultaneous video recording.

a First stage: the barium contrast (1) just reaches the esophagus. For orientation note the mandible (2), hyoid (3), and vallecula (4).

Fig. 9.33 b, c

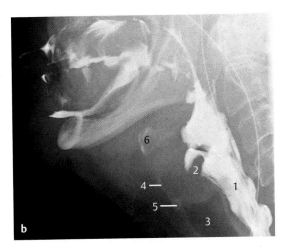

b Second stage: the contrast is located mainly in the hypopharynx and cervical esophagus (1). At this stage, the position of the epiglottis (2) should be horizontal (instead of vertical). However, the airways are closed and there is no extravasation of contrast medium in the larynx or trachea (3). The thyroid (4) and cricoid (5) cartilages are partly ossified and therefore visible. Note the elevation of the larynx and hyoid (6) in this phase.

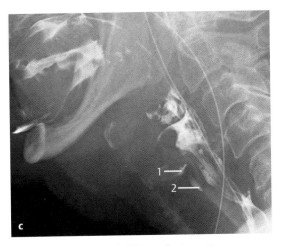

c Third stage: at the end of the swallowing action, some contrast is visible in the glottic region (1) and the posterior wall of the trachea (2), indicative of aspiration, probably due to epiglottic dysfunction during closure.

Esophageal Passage Disorders

Differential Diagnosis
- See also previous section on swallowing problems.
- Acute obstructions without previous complaints are mostly due to foreign bodies.

Points of Evaluation
- Patients with removable dentures may lack oral sensory input regarding the size of their food. This may also happen with sharp foreign bodies, which may cause perforations of the esophagus.
- Anatomic structures such as the aortic arch or an aberrant right esophageal artery are demonstrated as persistent impressions without stasis of contrast.

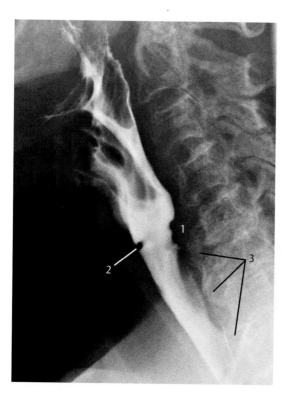

Fig. 9.34   Barium swallow, lateral view. Problems with esophageal passage can be a result of a variety of etiologies occurring either singly or in combination, such as neurologic coordination disorders, hypertrophy or spasms of the cricopharyngeal muscle (1), web formation (2), and osteophytic proliferations of the anterior cervical spine (3).

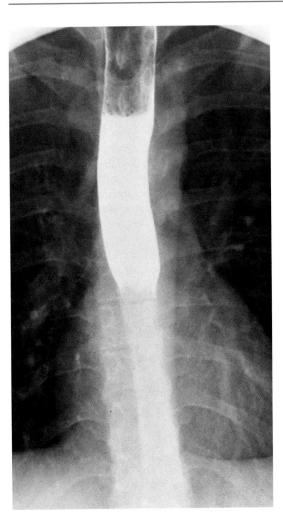

Fig. 9.35   Complete esophageal obstruction after dinner. Barium swallow. This patient had retrosternal compression and stasis of saliva after attempting to swallow a big piece of meat. The piece was stuck in the esophagus at mid-thoracic level and completely obstructed the passage of the contrast medium. There are no irregularities of the esophageal wall or signs of (unilateral) compression.

Zenker Diverticulum (1)

Differential Diagnosis

Large herniated laryngoceles from the supraglottic region through the thyrohyoid membrane might be demonstrated on CT or MRI as lesions with fluid levels, and could be confused with a Zenker diverticulum if no further swallowing evaluation is undertaken.

Points of Evaluation

Hypertrophy of the cricopharyngeal muscle may be the cause of a Zenker diverticulum, demonstrated by nonperistaltic contractions from the posterior side of the upper esophagus. Barium swallow shows the connection between the esophagus and a Zenker diverticulum, excluding other possible pathology. Large herniated laryngoceles will not fill with contrast during swallowing examination like a Zenker diverticulum, since they originate from the upper respiratory tract or larynx.

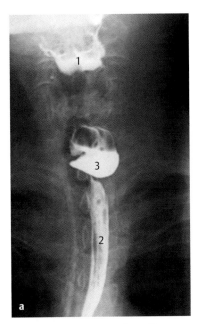
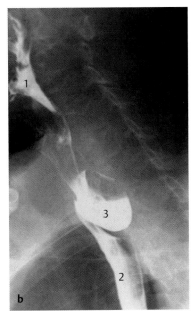

Fig. 9.36 a, b   Patients with swallowing problems and fetid regurgitation of food.

a Barium swallow, anteroposterior view.
After swallowing contrast, some contrast has remained in the hypopharynx (1) due to physiologic coating of the vallecula and piriform sinus. The majority of contrast has passed through the esophagus (2), but some contrast has accumulated in the diverticulum (3) situated below the entrance of the esophagus.

b Barium swallow, lateral view. This figure demonstrates passage of contrast from the oropharynx (1) to the distal esophagus (2), with stasis in the posteriorly located diverticulum (3). This so-called Zenker diverticulum is due to herniation through a weak part of the posterior pharyngeal wall, just above the cricopharyngeal muscle (Kilian triangle).

Zenker Diverticulum (2)

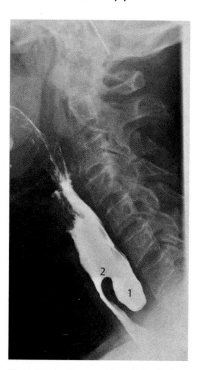

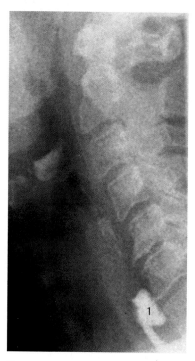

Fig. 9.37 Barium swallow, lateral view. Patient with a diverticulum (1) as long as the length of two cervical spine vertebra. Despite the more caudal position of the diverticulum in relation to the entrance of the trachea, sudden overflow of the contents of the diverticulum (2) into the esophagus carries a risk of aspiration.

Fig. 9.38 Barium swallow, lateral view. The evaluation of a diverticulum is occasionally more difficult, such as in this case with a small diverticulum (1) which might have been overlooked. Also, after surgical removal of a diverticulum, a small part of the rim might remain, which can still show some stasis of contrast or result in recurrence of the diverticulum.

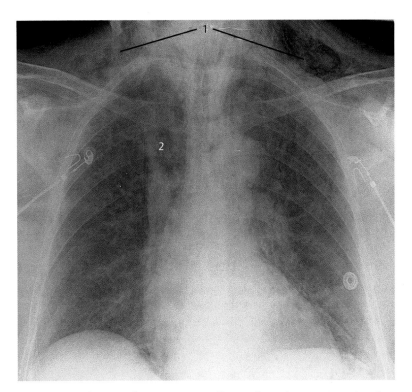

Fig. 9.39 Complications after treatment of Zenker diverticulum. Postoperative situation a few hours after laser treatment of a Zenker diverticulum. Because of retrosternal pain after surgery, the patient was suspected of having a perforation of the esophagus.

Chest radiograph, posteroanterior view. Air collections are observed in the subcutaneous lower neck tissues (1), particularly on the left side. Furthermore, the mediastinum is widened by dissection of air (2). There are no signs of pneumothorax. Progression of air entrapment and/or signs of mediastinitis must be monitored radiographically as well as clinically.

Laryngocele

Differential Diagnosis

- Laryngeal submucosal masses may be categorized as chondroid tumors, vascular tumors such as hemangiomas and paragangliomas, and submucosal cysts such as laryngocele, pharyngocele, thyroglossal duct cyst, and mucosal cyst.
- Less likely due to the location: branchial cleft cyst, Zenker diverticulum.

Points of Evaluation

- Laryngoceles are the result of an obstructed ventricular expansion into the paraglottic space. Most laryngoceles are internal, i.e., are restricted to the paraglottic space medial to the thyroid and hyoid. External laryngoceles expand through the thyrohyoid membrane. At levels superior to the hyoid, it is considered to be a pharyngocele. Small laryngoceles present with voice disorders (hoarseness) and respiratory problems (stridor). However, in cases of infection, symptoms progress rapidly and asphyxia may occur.
- The thyroglossal duct cyst is located in (or slightly off) the midline and related to the strap muscles. It may herniate posteriorly in the midline over the edge of the thyroid and be misinterpreted as a laryngocele.
- A branchial cleft cyst is situated medial to the great vessels.
- A Zenker diverticulum is located posterolateral to the esophagus at a lower level.

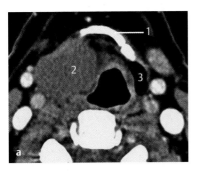
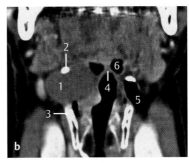

Fig. 9.40 a, b   Patient with hoarseness fluctuating.

a CT with intravenous contrast enhancement, axial. The axial slice at the lower border of the hyoid (1) reveals a homogeneous, expanding mass (2) on the right side, compromising the supralaryngeal airway on its medial side. Laterally, the mass seems to be extending through the thyrohyoid membrane. On the left side is an air space (3), which could be misinterpreted a part of the supralaryngeal lumen, but it is continuous with a newly formed space at lower levels. There is no contrast enhancement or calcification, excluding vascular or chondroid tumors.

b CT with intravenous contrast enhancement, coronal. The coronal view shows the mass on the right side (1) to be located between the hyoid (2) and thyroid (3) cartilages, confirming penetration of the thyrohyoid membrane. Note the epiglottis (4) and the vocal cords slightly below on both sides. These findings are suggestive of an internal and external laryngocele originating from the laryngeal ventricle and extending into the paraglottic space. Due to the presence of a malignancy in this area, this laryngocele was obstructed and thus had expanded in volume due to the fluid. On the left side, the previously mentioned air-filled space (5) is not continuous with the supralaryngeal space (6). It seems to follow the same course as the laryngocele on the right side, and must be considered to be a primary internal and external laryngocele of unknown etiology.

Pneumothorax

Differential Diagnosis
Beside surgical complications, pneumothorax may also arise after (minor) trauma or extensive coughing.

Points of Evaluation
Most cases of pneumothorax are much smaller than in the picture shown here, and most of them are located at the lung apex.

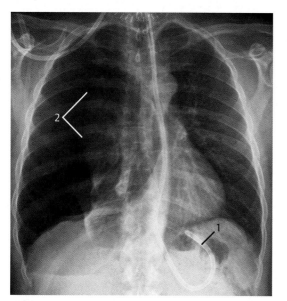

Fig. 9.41 Conventional radiography is used in positioning devices, such as intubation tubes or nasogastric feeding tubes, especially in cases of difficult positioning in cancer patients. In this case, the patient underwent laryngectomy a few days previously.

Chest radiograph, posteroanterior view. A nasogastric feeding tube (1) is positioned correctly in the stomach. The radiograph was taken for evaluation of progressive dyspnea. A pneumothorax on the right side was diagnosed with a severely collapsed lung (lateral border indicated: 2). An aspiration system was inserted and the normal position of the lung was restored within a few days.

Paralysis of the Recurrent Laryngeal Nerve

Differential Diagnosis

- Common etiologies revealed by the medical history are thoracic and thyroid gland surgical interventions, which may be radiographically confirmed by the presence of radiopaque clips.
- Benign compressive (schwannoma, paraganglioma) or infiltrative malignant lesions in the neck, such as primary tumors, metastases, lymphoma, thyroid disorders. Intrathoracic pathology such as aneurysms of the aortic arch or malignancies in the upper lung regions.

Points of Evaluation

- Clinical history and evaluation must be combined with a thorough radiographic evaluation of the complete course of the vagal and recurrent laryngeal nerve starting from the brainstem, through the jugular foramen in the skull base and its passage through the carotid sheath and upper thoracic cavity (aortic arch and right subclavian artery). MRI or CT may be used for this purpose.
- For illustrations of the above-mentioned pathologies, see other sections.

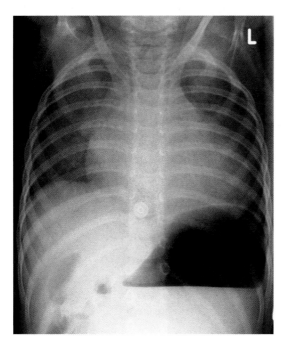

Fig. 9.42 A 7-year-old child with hoarseness and left vocal cord paralysis. Chest radiograph, posteroanterior view. The grossly dilated heart is compressing the recurrent laryngeal nerve against the aortic arch, resulting in dysfunction and left vocal cord paralysis. This phenomenon is not always recognized as a cause of recurrent nerve palsy.

Foreign Bodies

Some patients with psychiatric disorders often swallow all kinds of materials (e.g., spoons). Once these have passed through the esophagus and stomach, natural evacuation is almost certain. Even sharp needles are almost always passed without harm although the patient's clinical condition must be monitored and, as in most cases, radiologic investigations may be needed to reassure the patient (and sometimes the physician).

Differential Diagnosis
In case of suspicion of foreign bodies, stasis of saliva indicates complete obstruction of the esophagus. For accurate localization of radiopaque foreign bodies, radiography must be performed in several directions to exclude positioning outside the esophagus.

Points of Evaluation
In case of chronic inclusions or sharp foreign bodies, beware of migration to structures outside the esophagus with the risk of complications to nerves and vessels, and infections such as pneumonia and mediastinitis.

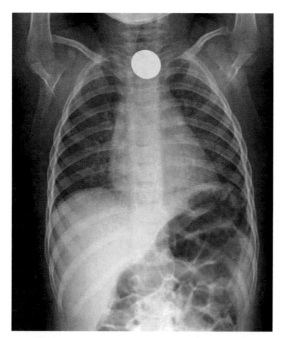

Fig. 9.43 Conventional radiography can still be convenient for evaluation of radiopaque foreign bodies, as in this 2-year-old child, who was suspected of swallowing a coin. Chest radiograph, posteroanterior view. A rounded density with a diameter of 21 mm was observed, equivalent to a 5 eurocent coin, which was seen to be a Dutch coin on removal. This position corresponds to the region of the hypopharynx or the upper esophageal sphincter.

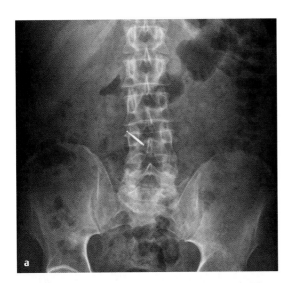

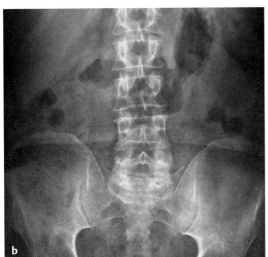

Fig. 9.44 a, b It may be somewhat unusual to end this ENT book with a radiograph of the pelvis. However, a physician always has to keep in mind the whole patient. This patient visited a dentist and accidentally swallowed a dental bur during treatment.

a, b Plain abdominal film, anteroposterior view. Fig. 9.44 a, taken one day after the incident, shows the radiopaque bur in the central abdomen, most probably in the jejunum. One week later (**b**), the bur had passed out of the body naturally.

Index